BODIES ACROSS BORDERS

Bodies Across Borders
The Global Circulation of Body Parts, Medical Tourists and Professionals

Edited by

BRONWYN PARRY
King's College London, UK

BETH GREENHOUGH
University of Oxford, UK

TIM BROWN AND ISABEL DYCK
Queen Mary University of London, UK

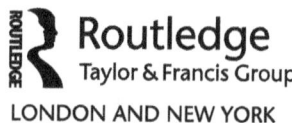

Routledge
Taylor & Francis Group

LONDON AND NEW YORK

First published 2015 by Ashgate Publishing

Published 2016 by Routledge
2 Park Square, Milton Park, Abingdon, Oxon OX14 4RN
711 Third Avenue, New York, NY 10017, USA

First issued in paperback 2017

Routledge is an imprint of the Taylor & Francis Group, an informa business

British Library Cataloguing in Publication Data
A catalogue record for this book is available from the British Library

The Library of Congress has cataloged the printed edition as follows:
Parry, Bronwyn.
  Bodies across borders : the global circulation of body parts, medical tourists and professionals / by Bronwyn Parry, Beth Greenhough, Tim Brown and Isabel Dyck.
    pages cm
  Includes bibliographical references and index.
  ISBN 978-1-4094-5717-6 (hardback)
  1. Medical tourism. 2. Medical tourism--Economic aspects. 3. Organ trafficking.
  4. Medical care. I. Greenhough, Beth. II. Brown, Tim. III. Dyck, Isabel. IV. Title.
  RA793.5.P37 2015
  362.1--dc23
                                                                        2014042800

ISBN 13: 978-1-138-30838-1 (pbk)
ISBN 13: 978-1-4094-5717-6 (hbk)

Contents

PART I: CORPOREAL CIRCULATIONS

PART II: TRANSNATIONAL BIO-MEDICAL TOURISM

PART III: MIGRATING MEDICAL EXPERTISE

PART IV: REGULATING BODIES ACROSS BORDERS

List of Figures and Tables

Figures

Tables

Notes on Contributors

Stephen Bach is professor of employment relations, Department of Management, King's College London. Stephen's principal research activities relate to public service HRM and changing workforce roles. His research interests include: international migration of health professionals; new ways of working in the public services; human resource management in the health sector; and the future of public service trade unions. His work has been published in the *British Journal of Industrial Relations, Human Relations* and *Work, Employment and Society*. His books include: *Employment Relations and the Health Service* (Routledge, 2004) and he is co-author of *The Modernisation of the Public Services and Employee Relations* (Palgrave Macmillan, 2012, with Ian Kessler). He is co-editor of *Managing Human Resources* (Wiley, 2013, with Martin Edwards).

Tim Brown is a senior lecturer in the School of Geography, Queen Mary University of London. His research has explored how ideas of risk and responsibility are articulated as technologies of self-care in contemporary public health discourse. More recently, he has applied the critical insights developed in this research into other areas; notably, global health and food security and environment and health in late-Victorian London. In addition to publishing widely in this area he co-edited *A Companion to Health and Medical Geography* (Wiley-Blackwell, 2009), was associate editor for health geography for *The Wiley-Blackwell Encyclopedia of Health, Illness, Behavior, and Society* (Wiley-Blackwell, 2014) and he is currently working on *Health Geographies: A Critical Introduction* (Wiley-Blackwell, 2015, with Andrews, Cummins, Greenhough and Power). He is on the editorial board of *Health & Place*.

Ruth Chadwick is professor of bioethics at the University of Manchester. From 2002–2013 she directed the ESRC Centre for Economic and Social Aspects of Genomics (Cesagen) at Cardiff University. She co-edits *Bioethics* and *Life Sciences, Society and Policy*, and she is a member of the Council of the Human Genome Organisation. She has also served on the Panel of Eminent Ethical Experts of the Food and Agriculture Organisation of the United Nations (FAO), and the UK Advisory Committee on Novel Foods and Processes (ACNFP). She is academician of the Academy of Social Sciences and fellow of the Learned Society of Wales, Hastings Center, New York; of the Royal Society of Arts; and of the Society of Biology. In 2005, she won the World Technology Network Award for Ethics.

Glenn Cohen is a professor at Harvard Law School and director of the Petrie-Flom Center for Health Law Policy, Biotechnology, and Bioethics at Harvard Law School. Professor Cohen is one of the world's leading experts on the intersection of bioethics (sometimes also called 'medical ethics') and the law, as well as health law. He also teaches civil procedure. From Seoul to Krakow to Vancouver, professor Cohen has spoken at legal, medical and industry conferences around the world and his work has been covered on ABC, PBS, NPR, in the *Boston Globe*, *Mother Jones*, and several other media venues. He is the author of more than 60 articles and chapters and his award-winning work has appeared in leading legal (including the *Stanford*, *Cornell*, and *Southern California Law Reviews*), medical (including the *New England Journal of Medicine, JAMA*), bioethics (including the *American Journal of Bioethics* and the *Hastings Center Report*) and public health (the *American Journal of Public Health*) journals, as well as Op-Eds in the *The New York Times* and *The Washington Post*. Cohen is the author of *Patients with Passports: Medical Tourism, Law, and Ethics* (Oxford University Press, 2014), the editor of *The Globalization of Health Care: Legal and Ethical Issues* (Oxford University Press, 2013), the co-editor of *Human Subjects Research Regulation: Perspectives on the Future* (MIT Press, 2014), with three other books under contract. Prior to becoming a professor he served as a law clerk to Judge Michael Boudin of the US Court of Appeals for the First Circuit and as a lawyer for US Department of Justice, Civil Division, Appellate Staff, where he handled litigation in the Courts of Appeals and (in conjunction with the Solicitor General's Office) in the US Supreme Court. Cohen was selected as a Radcliffe Institute Fellow for the 2012–2013 year and by the Greenwall Foundation to receive a Faculty Scholar Award in Bioethics. He is currently one of the key co-investigators on a multi-million award from the NFL Player's Association to protect and improve the health of NFL Members. He also leads the Ethics and Law initiative as part of the multi-million dollar NIH funded Harvard Catalyst, the Harvard Clinical and Translational Science Center program. He is also one of three editors-in-chief of the *Journal of Law and the Biosciences*, a peer-reviewed journal published by Oxford University Press.

John Connell is professor of human geography in the School of Geosciences, University of Sydney. He was previously at the Institute of Development Studies, University of Sussex, and the Department of Economics, Research School of Pacific Studies, ANU. He has been a consultant to the ILO, the WHO, the South Pacific Commission, the South Pacific Regional Environmental Program and the Asian Development Bank. His research interests cover development in the Pacific island region, the global/regional migration of health workers and the development of medical tourism. He has written more than 300 articles and over 20 books. The books include *Migration from Rural Areas: The Evidence from Village Studies* (with M. Lipton, R. Laishley and B. Dasgupta); *The Last Colonies* (with R. Aldrich); *Urbanisation in the Island Pacific. Towards Sustainable Development* (with J. Lea); *Sound Tracks: Popular Music, Identity and Place* (with C. Gibson); *The Global Health Care Chain. From the Pacific to the World*; *Medical Tourism*; and *Islands at Risk*.

Isabel Dyck is professor emerita in the School of Geography, Queen Mary University of London. She has published widely on the inter-relationships among the body, health, place and culture, and in her teaching explores the production of global health inequalities. Her research in Canada and the UK has investigated various settlement issues for international migrants, including health care and the re-making of home. Other recent work has examined the construction and practice of care relationships in long-term home health care. She has served on a number of editorial boards, including *Health & Place*.

Sheba George was awarded her MA and PhD degrees in sociology from the University of California at Berkeley. Since completing her doctorate, Dr George has consulted on research projects for Kaiser Permanente's Division of Research, and completed a NIMH AIDS research training postdoctoral fellowship in the Sociology Department at UCLA. Dr George's research broadly focuses on health inequities among underserved populations, using qualitative and mixed methods, particularly in the areas of health information technologies and healthcare workforce issues. She is the published author of two books by the University of California Press and several peer-reviewed articles. In her 2005 sole-authored book titled *When Women Come First: Gender and Class in Transnational Migration* (University of California Press, 2005), she examines the immigration and settlement experiences of Indian nurses to the United States and the transnational ties that keep them connected to their sending community in India. Furthermore, she see seeks to understand the barriers and facilitators to the provision of excellent care by international health care providers for their multicultural patients in inner-city US hospitals. She is adjunct associate professor at UCLA's Fielding School of Public Health, in the Department of Community Health Sciences.

Beth Greenhough is senior lecturer in geography at Queen Mary University of London. Her research draws on a combination of political-economic geography, cultural geography and science studies to explore the social implications of scientific innovations in the areas of health, biomedicine and the environment. Her current research interests include geographies of health and the biosciences, the global circulation of bodily commodities, the spaces of medical research, public health practice and environment-society relations, and her work has been funded by the AHRC, Barts and the London Charity Trust, the Brocher Foundation, ESRC and the Wellcome Trust. She has written extensively on the production and circulation of bodily commodities and human subjects, human-virus relations and bioethics.

Tamra Lysaght has a PhD from the University of Sydney in the history and philosophy of science. Her research interests focus on the bioethical, social and policy issues surrounding contested areas of science and emergent technologies, such as stem cell research and somatic cell nuclear transfer. She is currently a research fellow at the Centre for Biomedical Ethics at the National University of

Singapore, working on numerous ethics projects that address mental illness, whole genome sequencing, reproductive tissue donation and regenerative medicine.

Alan O'Connor is a barrister practising in Ireland. He worked as a research assistant in the ESRC Centre for Economic and Social Aspects of Genomics (Cesagen) in Cardiff University from 2011 to 2013 and maintains an active interest in bioethics and the ethics of legal practice.

Bronwyn Parry is an economic and cultural geographer who is now professor of social science, health and medicine at King's College London. She has written extensively on the rise and operation of the life sciences industries and on the commodification of bodily parts and bioinformation (*Trading the Genome: Investigating the Commodification of Bio-information*). She explored the social, ethical and legal complexities of biobanking and public attitudes to bodily donation through a three-year ethnography of the Addenbrooke's Hospital brain bank, work that culminated in a ground-breaking interactive public exhibition with the artist Ania Dabrowska and a book entitled *Mind Over Matter* completed in 2011. Bronwyn was a fellow of the Nuffield Council on Bioethics from 2007–2103 contributing to reports on the forensic use of bioinformation, the recent crisis in public health in the UK and dementia care. She has also undertaken comparative work on intellectual property regimes acting as a consultant for the UN and the UK governments in this capacity and sits on the editorial board of *Economy and Society*. She is currently undertaking a major Wellcome Trust-funded international bioethics project that investigates the production, consumption and regulation of assisted reproductive services in rural and urban India.

Guido Pennings obtained his PhD in moral sciences at the Free University Brussels (Belgium) with a thesis on the ethical aspects of medically assisted reproduction with donor gametes. He is professor of ethics and bioethics at Ghent University (Belgium) where he is also the director of the Bioethics Institute Ghent (BIG). In addition, he is affiliate lecturer in the Faculty of Politics, Psychology, Sociology and International Studies at Cambridge University and guest professor on 'Ethics in Reproductive Medicine' at the Faculty of Medicine and Pharmaceutical Sciences of the Free University Brussels. He is a member of the Ad Hoc Ethics Committee of the Centre for Reproductive Medicine of the Academic Hospital of the Free University Brussels, the Task Force on Ethics and Law of the European Society of Human Reproduction and Embryology (ESHRE), the National Advisory Committee on Bioethics and the Federal Commission on Research on Embryos in vitro.

Ingrid Schneider, PhD, is a senior researcher at the Research Centre on Biotechnology, Society, and the Environment (BIOGUM), in the Research Group on Medicine, and reader at the Department of Political Science, both at the University of Hamburg (Germany). She earned her PhD with a thesis on fetal tissue transplantation in 1996. Her habilitation thesis in political science (2010) covers the governance of the European patent system and analyses the EU's biotechnology patent directive (98/44/EC) and its implementation in the EU's member states. She has written extensively on technology assessment, biopolitics, legal regulation, transnational governance, property and personality rights on the human body, and on intellectual property rights. Since 1996 she has served in several advisory bodies for the German, Austrian and European Parliaments and for governmental agencies on embryo research, stem cells, transplantation, medical tourism, tissue economies, and other topics. She was a member of the Standing Advisory Committee before the European Patent Office (SACEPO) (2009–2012). In 2013 she was appointed by the European Commission as a member of the 'Expert Group on the development and implications of patent law in the field of biotechnology and genetic engineering'. In 2014, she was guest professor at the Life-Science-Governance Research Platform in the Department of Political Science of the University of Vienna.

Douglas Sipp graduated from Rutgers University in 1991 with a degree in English literature. After working in the software and publishing industries, he joined the RIKEN Center for Developmental Biology as head of the CDB communications office in 2002. From 2009 to 2014, he led a research unit studying policy and ethics issues in the translation and commercialization of stem cell research. He has published more than 40 research papers, reviews and book chapters, presented his work at dozens of international meetings, and has been extensively interviewed by the international scientific and mass media. He serves on task forces addressing the problem of the marketing of unproven stem cell treatments for both the International Society of Stem Cell Research and the International Society for Cell Therapy. He serves as managing editor for the journals *Zoological Science* and the *International Journal of Hematology*, and as business manager of the International Society for Developmental Biology and the Asia-Pacific Developmental Biology Network.

Leigh Turner is an associate professor at the University of Minnesota's Center for Bioethics, School of Public Health, and College of Pharmacy. Before joining the University of Minnesota faculty in 2008, Turner was associate professor and William Dawson Scholar in the Biomedical Ethics Unit at McGill University. From 1998–2000 Turner was assistant professor at the University of Toronto Joint Centre for Bioethics and clinical ethicist at Baycrest Centre for Geriatric Care and Sunnybrook and Women's College Health Sciences Centre. Turner has held visiting appointments at several institutions. In 2006–2007 Turner was distinguished visiting fellow at the Munk Centre for International Studies, University of Toronto. From 2003 to 2004 Turner was a member of the School of Social Science at the Institute for Advanced Study in Princeton, NJ. In 1999, Turner was visiting scholar at the Institute for the Medical Humanities, University of Texas Medical Branch. Turner's current research examines ethical issues related to international medical travel and the emergence of a global marketplace in health services. His research programme includes ethical and social analysis of 'medical tourism', cross-border commercial organ transplantation, the establishment of bioeconomies in East Asia, global migration of health care providers, and international trade in health services.

Wannes Van Hoof obtained an MA in philosophy and an MA in anthropology from the Catholic University Leuven and a PhD in philosophy from Ghent University with a thesis on ethical problems related to cross-border reproductive care. He is currently working at the Bioethics Institute Ghent (BIG). As an empirical bioethicist, his research focuses on the ethics of infertility treatment and the experiences of cross-border patients.

Sallie Yea is an assistant professor of geography at the National Institute of Education, Nanyang Technological University, Singapore. Before that she held positions at NUS (geography) and RMIT University (international development). Sallie has been researching issues of vulnerable mobilities, unfree labour and human trafficking since 2002. She has published widely on these topics in journals such as *Environment and Planning D*, *Gender, Place & Culture*, and *Singapore Journal of Tropical Geography*. She recently edited a volume *Human Trafficking in Asia: Forcing Issues* (Routledge, 2014) and *Women Trafficking in Korea* (Routledge, 2014). Her current research focuses on two topics: commercial organ provision in Asia; and unfree labour in Asia's long haul fishing industry and amongst male migrant workers in Singapore.

Preface

The inspiration for this edited collection was a two day workshop 'Bodies across Borders' hosted by the Fondation Brocher at their centre near Geneva, Switzerland, in December 2010. The workshop was organised by the editors of the collection, at the time all members of the *Health, Place and Society* research theme of the School of Geography, Queen Mary University of London.

The rationale for the workshop was the recognition that the fields of medicine and healthcare are being transformed by new communications and biomedical technologies, which have facilitated marked increases in the global circulation of body parts, patients and medical professionals across international borders. These movements often echo other movements of capital and resources, travelling from rural to urban areas, from poor to rich, and from the global South to the global North.

This edited collection builds on the intensive and highly productive discussion that took place over the course of those two days in December by drawing together a number of important contributions on three inter-related areas: bodily commodities, biomedical tourism and the migration of health care professionals. The aim of the collection, as with the workshop, is to elucidate the common themes, concerns and issues of relevance to those whose work either addresses or is affected by the global circulation of bodies across borders.

Our sincerest thanks go to the Fondation Brocher for funding and organising what was a very successful workshop, to the presenters for offering such insightful papers and to the participants for their invaluable input to the discussion. Our sincerest thanks also go to those presenters and other authors who agreed to contribute to this collection. Special thanks to Ashgate, and in particular Valerie Rose, for being so flexible and for guiding us through the long process from proposal to manuscript completion.

Bronwyn Parry, Beth Greenhough, Tim Brown and Isabel Dyck, 2014

Acknowledgements

This book was inspired by the lively discussions between participants at the Brocher Foundation workshop on Bodies Across Borders in December 2010. The authors would like to acknowledge the support of the Brocher Foundation for both this book and for sponsorship of the workshop upon which this volume is based. The Brocher Foundation's mission is to encourage research on the ethical, legal, social and economic implications of new medical technologies. Its main activities are to host visiting researchers and to organise symposia, workshops and summer academies. More information about the Brocher Foundation programme is available at: www.brocher.ch. The authors would also like to thank the School of Geography, Queen Mary University of London, for their support.

Chapter 1

Introduction

Bronwyn Parry, Beth Greenhough, Tim Brown and Isabel Dyck

Introduction

The fields of medicine and healthcare, historically organised at a local or national scale, are being radically transformed by new communication, transport and biotechnologies that facilitate the creation of a genuinely globalised sphere of biomedical production and consumption. This emerging market is characterised by the circulation of bodily materials, patients and expertise across what have traditionally been relatively secure ontological and geographical borders. Bodily parts that were once functionally non-transferable (for example tissues, organs and genetic information) are now capable of being sustained across space and time, available to be re-incorporated within other failing bodies or employed commercially as economically generative resources within burgeoning global life science industries. Individuals with the inclination and financial capacity now, similarly, have unprecedented opportunities to travel internationally to seek out the bodily resources and medical expertise necessary to make their goal of corporeal regeneration a success. The servicing of these desires is equally drawing medical personnel to, and from, their respective countries of origin towards global hubs of biomedical expertise, while the opportunity to 'outsource' therapeutic and compassionate labour that was once thoroughly 'domesticated' is everyday creating vibrant new economies in 'offshored care'.

While the global circulation of bodily commodities, medical tourists and healthcare workers has been the subject of some research to date, this work is often disparately located within disciplinary fields and specialisms. Policy responses to different aspects of the globalisation of medicine similarly target specific interventions and issues (such as the UK strategy of sending NHS patients abroad for treatment to help reducing waiting lists (Hanna et al., 2009), while published reports and factsheets examine trends in isolation, as evidenced by recent global reports on organ trafficking (Nullis-Kapp, 2004); medical tourism (Chinai and Goswami, 2007) and the migration of health workers (WHO, 2010). As academic and policy debates tend to focus on particular issues and perspectives there is little opportunity for scholars, policy makers and professionals in medicine and healthcare to share insights into the different ways in which bodies cross national borders, or to explore the overarching ethical, legal or social implications of the acceleration of bodily circulations within this emergent political economy of globalised biomedical healthcare. This book draws together a number of important contributions from acknowledged leaders in these three respective fields (bodily commodities, medical tourism and the migration of health care professionals) with a view to elucidating the common themes, concerns and issues of relevance to those whose work either addresses, or is affected by, the global circulation of bodies across borders. The book explores and maps out the key characteristics of this emerging, although as yet poorly researched global trade, paying particular attention to the social and spatial dynamics of this transactional economy. These typically echo those that attend the circulation of other forms of capital and resources in contemporary society: travelling from rural to urban areas, from poor to rich and from the Global South to the Global North (Scheper-Hughes, 2000). It poses a series of key, crosscutting questions designed to illuminate the cultural, ethical and legal implications of the dynamics of this circulation of bodies across borders. These include: i) How, where and why do bodies cross borders? ii) How does the global circulation of bodies and body-parts impact on healthcare services? iii) How are and should the circulation of bodies across borders, in the service or pursuit of medicine and healthcare, be regulated?

Part I (Corporeal Circulations) builds on an existing body of academic scholarship (see, for example, Scheper-Hughes and Wacquant, 2002; Waldby and Mitchell, 2006) that has explored the emergence of new global economies in bodily commodities. Much of this work has focused on the question of how different kinds of bodily materials, from gametes to fresh kidneys, are circulated internationally and under what terms and conditions. Particular attention has been paid to examining how changes in the constitution of such materials – from embodied organs to extracted tissues, sequenced DNA or bioinformation – affects how they can then be utilised as resources (for example as components of new manufactured technologies such as stem cell lines) and how this, in turn, shapes how they enter the market: be it as gifts, commodities or alienable forms of property (Parry, 2004).

One of the most developed set of literatures in this field concerns bio and tissue banking. Here scholars have drawn attention to concerns about the ways in which such samples are collected and made available as economic as well as scientific resources (Parry, 2008; Greenhough, 2006). Chapter 2 by Chadwick and O'Connor extends these debates by examining the specific issues associated with the transportation of biobanked materials across national borders, highlighting how the movement of these materials differs from the other forms of circulation considered in this volume. They argue that the trajectories of the materials banked by tissue donors are distinct from those made by prospective patients and medical professionals as they are not self-directed. Donors to biobanks arguably lack both autonomy and agency, having, effectively, no say and no control over how their samples will be used, or by whom. Chadwick and O'Connor highlight some of the challenges that arise when seeking to protect the interests of donors across international and regulatory boundaries, including protecting the interests and confidentiality (where requested) of donors, and addressing the inequalities that may arise between those who provide biobanked material (particularly those in less developed economies) and those who benefit from its exploitation. They also propose some useful ways forward, including proposals to enhance the role of contractual agreements between donating and receiving nations and enterprises; cross-border harmonisation of regulations (something also explored later in this volume in relation to medical tourism) and a complementary harmonisation of ethical values.

Yea's following Chapter 3 highlights the key role that cultural, moral, social and economic factors play in shaping the contexts within which human body parts are circulated through the burgeoning global organ trade. Her analysis of the experiences of economically marginalised male Filipino kidney donors/sellers does not seek to deny the exploitative nature of this trade, but simultaneously works to refute the now commonplace tendency in the international media, and in some academic papers, to portray such donors as simply 'victims'. Where Chadwick and O'Connor draw our attention to the lack of control that biobank donors have in dictating how their bodily commodities are used Yea highlights how these Filipino men reclaim some degree of agency, if not over the use of their organs, then at least over the way in which they, as donors, are characterised in the public domain. As she carefully details, they exert their agency by challenging their identification as 'victims' of organ trafficking with discourses that assert their role as both male breadwinners and 'heroes' who have suffered and sacrificed their vitality for the good of their families and dependants. Yea's focus on Filipino men who remain at home also provides an interesting counterpoint to other studies that focus on the experiences of Filipino nurses who have migrated abroad to meet the demands of the ever expanding global North healthcare sector (Choy, 2003).

Like Chadwick and O'Connor, Parry in Chapter 4 explores the global variation that exists in approaches to regulation of biobanks but she does so in order to demonstrate how this heterogeneity provides the conditions for the establishment of a highly variegated international marketplace for human sperm. In order to explore why the United States seems to be dominating this emerging market she begins by analysing how the global circulation of reproductive materials first became possible, paying particular attention to the historiography of the development of its usage as a bankable commodity. Like both Yea and Chadwick and O'Connor, she demonstrates how significant aspects of globalisation have been in facilitating the technological and commercial development of this trade. Alongside this, however, like Yea, she also explores how aspects of this trade are represented and socially constructed. Drawing analogies with practices of selective breeding, husbandry and pedigree in agriculture she demonstrates how sperm donors are 'characterised', a performative act that plays a key role in 'singularising' them in relation to their competitors in such a way that they are favourably evaluated and judged as preferable. Parry voices concerns about the nature of these representations, suggesting that part of the implicit work of donor profiling is to create new technologies and devices that construct and embed wider societal norms of what counts as 'good' and 'bad' stock and to separate them one from the other. Whilst this can be viewed simply as a technique for maximising healthy conception, it can also, she argues, have more troubling implications invoking the spectre of eugenics and its belief in the need to engineer for better 'population quality'.

Part II (Transnational Bio-medical Tourism) examines the transnational movement of patients across borders as part of the recent dramatic rise in medical tourism. There has been some debate as to what distinguishes medical tourism from other forms of health travel, such as a visit to a health spa or retreat, with some authors (see, for example, Turner and Schneider, this volume) suggesting that the term 'tourism' perhaps trivialises the often serious and complex medical procedures undergone by patients and should, more rightfully, be revoked in favour of more accurate terms such as cross-border care or medical travel. The billing of places as glamorous global health destinations or 'health theme parks' (see Connell, this volume) sits uncomfortably beside Turner's (this volume) reminder of the very serious and complicated nature of many of the procedures there undertaken and the risks involved for these purported 'tourists'.

It is difficult to find accurate numbers to map the growth in patients travelling abroad for medical treatment, but the rapid increase in the number and size of facilities in the top medical tourism destination countries, including Thailand, Malaysia, India, Singapore, The Philippines and Mexico (Connell, 2006; Turner, 2007), reflects how medical travel has changed from being dominated by local cross-border movements, or journeys made by expatriates returning 'home' for medical treatment to a genuinely global industry. Amongst others influences, the growth in medical tourism has been driven by three key factors: the rise in the internet which has facilitated the direct marketing and promotion of medical tourism destinations to patients (Lunt and Carrera, 2011; Connell, this volume); the growth in medical tourism intermediaries (Turner, this volume), who, not unlike the kidney brokers described by Yea, have actively expedited the movement of bodies across borders; and the support and investment provided by governments in destination countries who see medical tourism as a growth industry and an important source of foreign direct investment (Ormond and Mainil, 2014).

The chapters in this volume explore some of the challenges posed by medical tourism, including the impacts of this growth industry on host and destination countries and the differences in expectations and standards of care that emerge when patients cross national borders. The transnational healthcare industry has sharpened disparities in access between, for example, the private foreign patients who increasingly utilise the new state-of-the-art hospitals provided for them, and the majority of the domestic population who are consigned to the remaining very poorly resourced local public health services (see for example Chinai and Goswami's 2007 report on India). Critics point to the diversion of both public funds and skilled personnel towards the medical tourism industry. This context informs Connell's critical overview of the medical tourism industry in Chapter 5 in which he highlights how its development reflects broader trends in post-industrial societies, including the privatisation and globalisation of healthcare and the emergence of the patient 'consumer' with a robust sense of entitlement to physical and biological perfection.

For Connell, patients remain, for the most part, the beneficiaries of the emerging medical tourism industry. However, both Turner in Chapter 6, and Van Hoof and Pennings in Chapter 7, weigh the advantages of travelling abroad for medical care, including the opportunity to access services which are either inaccessible (due to, for example, long waiting lists or high costs) or illegal in the home country (for example fertility treatment for same sex couples), against what they perceive to be some of the significant disadvantages. In Chapter 6 Turner suggests that the profit-driven nature of the medical tourism sector puts patients at risk of being encouraged to opt for procedures that may be unnecessary, which may not meet leading international standards of health care provision (leading to a greater risk of complications and infection) and about which they may be poorly informed. Furthermore, once the procedure is completed, there are concerns about the provision (and cost) of post-operative care in the home country and legal redress should things go wrong. As a case in point in Chapter 7 Van Hoof and Pennings focus specifically on the issue of cross-border reproductive care, setting an appreciation of reproductive autonomy (as a human right) against concerns about safety, success rates and the possibility of legal redress, as well as highlighting some case-specific issues including the complications of obtaining citizenship for children born abroad using surrogate mothers and donor gametes (see also Schneider, this volume).

Part III (Migrating Medical Expertise) focuses on issues associated with the global circulation of medical professionals, knowledge and expertise. A global crisis in the health care labour force has been signalled in media coverage, policy bulletins and scholarly work with the World Health Organisation for some while, with the latter estimating a shortage of 4.3 million health care workers as early as 2006. While this category of 'health care worker' is broad, most attention has been paid to the migration of nurses, and to some extent doctors. A 'brain drain' from low-income countries is of particular concern. While nurses from the Philippines (110,000) and doctors from India (56,000) constitute the largest share of the migrant health workforce in Organisation for Economic Cooperation and Development countries, the WHO (2010, n.p.) notes that 'countries with smaller populations than India and the Philippines may suffer from a larger impact in terms of expatriation rates. Over 50% of highly-trained health workers leave for better job opportunities abroad in some low-income countries'. A push-pull model in a global market where embodied medical expertise (doctors, nurses and other health care workers) is at a premium is commonly employed to explain and describe such movements. Rich countries providing higher salaries, training opportunities and better working conditions pull in workers, while poor working conditions and low remuneration in low-income and conflict-ridden countries push workers to other countries and world regions.

This migration is set within a global health worker labour market where health professionals comprise a flexible labour force moving to fill gaps while advancing personal interests and the economic goals of households. But individual and household decisions need to be located in global migration flows and their context.

Economic goals of nations, feminisation of the work force, demographic shifts, and work directives, such as EU working hours, all have an influence. While early migrations tended to follow the routes of colonial ties, this is largely superseded by economic movement and new geopolitical alignments (for overviews, see Dovlo, 2007; Kingma, 2007; and OECD, 2010). The UK, for example, has filled its long-standing gap in the domestic production of health professionals with health care workers from different regions of the world, with the most recent wave of recruitment targeting nurses from Eastern Europe (The Guardian, 2013). The Philippines incorporates the export of its nurses, as human capital, into its national economic strategy with remittances as a crucial source of income. As the largest global exporter of nurses it has long had more registered nurses working overseas than it does domestically (Ball, 2004). In sum, health worker migrants as skilled labour constitute an important commodity with exchange value in a global market.

Most literature and reports focus on the obvious concerns in relation to access to health care and health care provision in low ratio doctor to patient countries, and on ways to regulate flows of skilled health workers. Although this is difficult to monitor due to lack of systematic statistics, especially in the global South, progress has been made with attempts to retain staff through, for example, salary top ups, improved career structures and other measures, and a WHO code of conduct that actively discourages the poaching of nurses from crisis areas. While most work is at the macro level, some on nurses' experience has shown how individual stories of migration mesh with government policy revealing also the gendered and racialised dimensions of health care worker migration (Hardill and Macdonald, 2000; Ball, 2004).

Two chapters in Part III bring further depth to this field of study providing detailed analyses of the complex interweaving of economic and non-economic factors that facilitate and maintain migratory flows of skilled health worker migrants. The first of these is George's exploration of the experiences of Indian nurses in the US in Chapter 8; the second, Bach's analysis of the UK experience in Chapter 9. Bach notes that even in a context of enhanced global mobility and free movement of labour (in the case of the European movement), governments can still exert influence through immigration rules, licensing requirements and ethical recruitment codes. He traces three phases of state policy to illustrate the impacts of such regulations and their effects on migrant nurses' experiences. George similarly provides a nuanced ethnographic account of Indian nurses' experiences in the United States. This highlights the specific challenges faced by this group, notably the difficulties they experience being accepted as equals to their US peers. As she demonstrates, their pre-migration employment and training, differences in professional cultures, expectations around emotional labour and problems of trust together combine to create for them a highly racialised work environment and experience in the US context.

Part IV of the volume (Regulating Bodies Across Borders) is devoted to analysing the complex question of how, if at all, it might be possible to regulate the traffic of 'bodies across borders' in a globalised world. Both Cohen and Schnieder in Chapters 10 and 11 begin this task by focusing attention on the legal and ethical implications of extending medical care beyond the conventional parameters of the nation state and the profound complexities of attempting to create regulations that can secure the quality and efficacy of this care. Cohen's finely grained analysis of the filigree of domestic and international regulatory measures and international directives that interface to monitor and regulate the provision of health care across borders is particularly useful as it reveals the intricacy of the response that will be required to ensure that provision of care by offshore providers is both longitudinally cost effective but also, and relatedly, of sufficient quality.

His typology of the highly variegated plans that health insurance companies are offering their subscribers provides an important insight into the ways the global market for health care provision is likely to be articulated in the future and through which uptake of medical tourism is currently being incentivized. Significantly it also suggests points of entry for interventions, what Cohen calls 'channeling regimes', that can be employed to discipline the market by only directing prospective patients to those facilities with more robust accreditation; which would consent to international jurisdiction, or provide insurance in cases of medical malpractice.

Schneider reminds the reader of the diversity of the practices that have come to be encompassed by the term 'medical tourism', noting that these have included: travel for routinized medical care (such as hip replacements or dental work); the recruitment and migration of medical staff and health care workers; the acquisition and circulation of tissues, organs, stem cells and gametes used in advanced biomedicine; and even the outsourcing of clinical trials and the accessing of experimental treatments (such as preimplantation genetic diagnosis, surrogacy or stem cell therapies) that remain unlawful in the patients home country. The inherently extraterritorial nature of these practices stands in direct opposition to the thoroughly embedded nature of judicial law making which remains wedded (for the most part) to the concepts of sovereign rights and national jurisdictions. As she illustrates, whilst various instruments, such as criminal and civil law enforcement measures are available to those who wish to regulate the terms and conditions by which patients, providers, clinicians and researchers can access or develop care regimes, their effectiveness is ultimately constrained by the geographical limits of their legislative reach.

Both chapters clearly highlight a key challenge for regulators: that of how to generate commensurable information and universal metrics to determine quality of care that are based on objective indicators such as mortality, avoidable error and acquired infection rates rather than on more unreliable culturally inflected measures such as self-certification of standards. Whilst both Cohen and Schneider believe recent EU directives provide promising examples of how supranational regulation can be deployed to enhance the quality of cross border healthcare, patient trust and mobility, each suggests that the legality of some of these mechanisms remains in question. The most promising opportunities for the enhancement of regulation of medical tourism may lie, as Schneider argues in 'soft law' and in other horizontal forms of governance such as self- regulation within the industry (conditionalities imposed by health care insurance providers and standard setting for international benchmarks of professional conduct and best practice) that could ultimately provide normative frameworks for medical governance that have the capacity to transcend territorial borders.

All this, however, assumes that the object of regulation – this thing known as 'medical tourism' – remains stable and open to consistent classification. In the final chapter in this volume Lysaght and Sipp turn this presumption on its head with their incisive critique of current conceptualisations of what is described colloquially as 'stem cell tourism'. Whilst as they note, this practice has been casually conflated with others forms of cross border health care seeking behaviour – it in fact varies from them in ways that are significant both ontologically and in terms of regulatory practice. As they note, most studies of medical tourism assume that patients are seeking standardised care and thus direct their analysis to the quality of care offered by medical providers. The touristic aspects of their health seeking behaviour are emphasised and travel is assumed to be unidirectional: e.g. the patients are travelling to the provider. In the case of stem cell therapies, however, patients are seeking to access care that is not only experimental but also, in many jurisdictions, illegal. The inconsistency of approaches to the regulation of stem cell therapy has created a highly differentiated legal landscape. In this instance it proves to be providers (who range from clinicians to research scientists) who are 'shopping around' to exploit regulatory loopholes and niche locations in which to establish clinics whose presence would not elsewhere be tolerated.

Attempting to subject this kind of therapy to the same forms of regulatory control that Cohen and Schneider outline is deeply problematic due in part to the fact that the ontological status of these practices is so uncertain: does stem cell therapy constitute medical care, a scientific experiment or an unregulated clinical trial? Whilst its status remains so unstable the register in which regulation could or should operate remains similarly indistinct. What is evident though is that the continued concentration on the narrative of 'tourism', serves only as Lysaght and Sipp demonstrate, to focus attention on the most vulnerable actors in this scenario – desperately ill patients – rather than the clinics and providers whose legal culpabilities in providing such unlicensed, risky and illegal therapies far outweighs any that can be laid at the door of the medical 'tourist', so described.

In conclusion, we would like to suggest a number of cross-cutting themes that are highlighted by bringing together different examples of the movement of bodies across borders from diverse disciplinary perspectives. Firstly, the chapters in this volume highlight the challenges of tracing the movement of bodies across borders. Yea's need to draw on personal contacts to access Filipino men for her research on organ donors (see also Moniruzzaman, 2007), the lack of reliable figures on the number of patients travelling abroad for medical treatment (Connell; Turner, this volume) and the numbers of trained medical personal migrating from lesser to more developed nations, and the absence of commensurable information and universal metrics for evaluating medical tourism facilities all attest to the great difficulties of obtaining an accurate picture of the flows that characterize this new economy. Secondly, the chapters have drawn attention to the role that technology has played in facilitating the circulation of these new resources, commodities and consumers. Advancements in storage, transport and communication technologies that range from the cryogenic preservation methods that allow for the storage and global circulation of human (and bovine) gametes, to the internet, with its role in promoting medical tourism and experimental techniques (such as stem cell therapy, Lysaght and Sipp, this volume) which, in turn, motivate patients to cross international borders have all been key drivers of this new trade. Thirdly, these works have revealed the key role played in all the case studies by 'middle men' or brokers who have identified new lucrative forms of employment in arranging the movement of bodies across borders, matching Filipino kidney sellers with buyers and transplant surgeons, providing medical tourist packages incorporating flights, accommodation and even excursions with surgery, and sourcing medical staff from the global South to meet care demands in the global North (Santiago, 2010).

Fourthly, this volume highlights commensurabilities and differences in the ethical, legal and social issues raised by these movements. Striking, for example, is the balance between the demand for anonymity (to protect the privacy of biobank, sperm and kidney donors or the confidentiality of medical tourists) with the need to 'market' the pedigree of bodily commodities, be they bio information, sperm, kidneys, or the expertise of medical professionals and medical tourist services. Finally, we might consider how the capacity to move bodies across borders can shape our sense of self and the extent to which we, as humans, feel able to exert control over our bodies and their derivatives. Chadwick and O'Connor (this volume) stress biobank donors' lack of agency and control over what happens to their materials. Yea describes kidney sellers' attempts to retain some control over their representation in the media, if not their donated kidneys as a reclaiming of agency, although others would argue that these kidney donors are victims of forms of structural violence which make their decision to sell a kidney perhaps less autonomous than it seems (Sunder Rajan, 2007). Connell's chapter (this volume) highlights how, in contrast to the donor, the patient is reconfigured as a consumer who is entitled to the best health (and offspring) they can afford. Here the perfect healthy body increasingly becomes something that those who can afford the bodily commodities (e.g. stem cells or organ transplants or donors' eggs) and medical services (such as those provided by medical tourism destinations like Bumrungrad International Hospitial, Thailand) feel entitled to, reflecting how inequalities in economic wealth remain a key determinate of who is, and is not, ultimately in a position to benefit from the movement of bodies across borders.

References

Ball, R.E., 2004. Divergent Development, Racialised Rights: Globalised labour markets and the trade of nurses – the case of the Philippines. *Women's Studies International Forum*, 27, pp. 119–33.

Chinai, R. and Goswami, R., 2007. Medical Visas Mark Growth of Indian Medical Tourism. *Bulletin of the World Health Organization*, 85(3), pp. 161–244.

Choy, C.C., 2003. *Empire of Care: Nursing and migration in Filipino American history. American encounters/Global interactions*. Durham, NC: Duke University Press.

Connell, J., 2006, Medical Tourism: Sea, sun, sand and surgery. *Tourism Management*, 27, pp. 1093–100.

Dovlo, D., 2007. Migration of Nurse from Sub-Saharan Africa: A review of issues and challenges. *Health Services Research*, 42(3), pp. 1373–88.

Greenhough, B., 2006. Decontextualised? Dissociated? Detached? Mapping the networks of bioinformatics exchange. *Environment and Planning A*, 38, pp. 445–63.

Hanna, S.A., Saksena, J., Legge, S. and Ware, H.E., 2009. Sending NHS Patients for Operations Abroad: Is the holiday over? *Annals of the Royal College of Surgeons*, 91(2), pp. 128–30.

Hardill, I. and Macdonald, S., 2000. Skilled International Migration: The experience of nurses in the UK, *Regional Studies*, 34(7), pp. 681–92.

Kingma, M., 2007. Nurses on the Move: A global overview. *Health Services Research*, 42(3), pp. 1281–98.

Lunt, N. and Carrera, P., 2011. Advice for Prospective Medical Tourists: Systematic review of consumer sites. *Tourism Review*, 66(1/2), pp. 57–67.

Moniruzzaman, M., 2007. Underground Fieldwork with 33 Kidney Sellers in Bangladesh: Issues of access and methods. In: J.C. Cohen and B. Seaton, eds. 2007. *Comparative Program on Health and Society Working Paper Series 2006–2007*. Toronto: Munk Centre for International Studies, University of Toronto, pp. 83–108.

Nullis-Kapp, C., 2004. Organ Trafficking and Transplantation Pose New Challenges. *Bulletin of the World Health Organisation*, 82(9), p. 715.

OECD, 2010. Policy Brief: International migration of health workers. Paris: OECD.

Ormond, M. and Mainil, T., 2014. Government Strategies. In: N. Lunt, J. Hanefeld and D. Horsfall, eds. 2014. *Handbook on Medical Tourism and Patient Mobility*. London: Edward Elgar.

Parry, B., 2008. Entangled Exchange: Reconceptualising the characterisation and practice of bodily commodification. *Geoforum*, 39(3), pp. 1133–44.

Rose, H., 2001, *The Commodification of Bioinformation: The Icelandic health sector database*. London: The Wellcome Trust.

Santiago, L., 2010. Made for Canada, Product of the Philippines: Global nurse migrations and the geopolitics of global justice. Poster presented at the *Bodies Across Borders symposium*, Brocher Foundation, Geneva, December 2010.

Scheper-Hughes, N., 2000. The Global Traffic in Human Organs. *Current Anthropology*, 41, pp. 191–224.

Scheper-Hughes, N. and Wacquant, L., 2002. *Commodifying Bodies*. London: Sage.

Stilwell, B., Diallo, K., Zurn, P., Vujicic, M., Adams, A. and Dal Poz, M., 2004. Migration of Health-Care Workers from Developing Countries: Strategic approaches to its management. *Bulletin of the World Health Organization*, 82(8), pp. 559–636.

Sunder-Rajan, K., 2006. *Biocapital: The constitution of postgenomic life*. Durham, NC: Duke University Press.

The Guardian, 2013. Health: Third of trusts fill nurse shortfalls from abroad. *The Guardian* (14 October). [online] Available at: <http://www.theguardian.com/society/2013/oct/14/health-trusts-nurse-shortfalls-recruit-abroad> [Accessed 14 April 2014].

Turner, L., 2007. First World care at Third World Prices: Globalisation, bioethics and medical tourism. *Biosocieties*, 2, pp. 303–25.

Waldby, C. and Mitchell, R., 2006. *Tissue Economies*. Durham, NC: Duke University Press.

WHO, 2006. *Working Together for Health: The World Health Report 2006*. Geneva: World Health Organization.

———, 2006 (updated 2010). *Migration of Health Workers. Fact sheet no. 301*. [online] Available at: <http://www.who.int/mediacentre/factsheets/fs301/en/> [Accessed 14 April 2014].

PART I
Corporeal Circulations

Chapter 2

Biobanking Across Borders

Ruth Chadwick and Alan O'Connor

Introduction: Why Sample Exchange?

The development of national initiatives in biobanking in countries such as Iceland, Estonia and the UK has given rise to a great deal of social, legal and ethical discussion over the past decade and more. It is the possibilities of exchange at the international level, however, that have now moved centre stage. There are a number of contexts within which human tissue samples may be taken across borders. They may be sought out for a particular research project, they may be sent individually for clinical tests or, in the age of 'recreational' genetics, even gathered from across the world to establish baseline data to be tested against. They may also be brought to one place to assemble a biobank with samples from across the world to aid in general scientific research.

The exchange of human tissue samples across borders has led, first to arguments for the importance of exchange of samples and data, and second to debates about how to deal with potential problems that might arise from an ethical point of view. The argument for exchange goes as follows. Population wide biobank research is of potentially very great importance for future health care – for example, by finding out the genetic basis underlying the variation influencing our susceptibilities to common diseases and to adverse drug responses. To maximise its effectiveness, however, and achieve sufficient statistical power, collaboration between different initiatives is required. While the argument from statistical power is important, we shall not discuss this further here. The challenging ethical issues concern the potential difficulties arising out of sample transfer.

Transfer of Samples: The Challenges

The nub of the ethical debate arises from potential and actual differences in practice and procedures between different cultural contexts. This is particularly problematic in relation to transfer of samples from historical collections, where consent has been given to use within a particular setting, but also applies prospectively. Sample donors may consent to specific conditions, but it may not be possible for the donee institution to guarantee that these conditions will be observed in all settings. There may also be a qualitative difference between those cases where tissue samples are 'sent' by the initiating party and those where samples are 'sought'. The former may imply that the sample donor maintains a high level of control, setting the ground rules for how the sample may be used. Though in the latter case, the donor may not have any say over the subsequent use of their tissue.

Although differences in expectations of professional behaviour give rise to debates in other areas, for example, in what has come to be known as health care tourism, the issues are different: it is one thing for someone voluntarily to go to another setting for treatment, even if there are grounds for thinking it unwise; it is another for an institution to transfer a person's samples to a context where there is no control over how they may be used.

The issue of human embryonic stem cell (HESC) transfer is illustrative of some of the issues which arise. The moral nature of HESCs is disputed, as are questions around how cell lines should be obtained and used, and cultural norms may play a part in informing how the answers to these questions are arrived at (Salter and Salter, 2007). Issues have arisen about the origin of cell lines sought by researchers from abroad and the use to which samples sent away might be put. In these contexts, cultural understanding is necessary in order for each party to a transaction to satisfy their own ethical concerns. In the absence of trust in the ethical soundness of research, international collaborations may not be possible (Salter, 2008).

There are three particularly problematic areas in which issues arise: consent, data protection and benefit-sharing. These are summarised below. In the course of the subsequent discussion we will outline proposals at EU level for dealing with data transfer and a case study within the EU which proposed dealing with these issues by mechanisms of contract. We will then look at regulatory approaches within the EU and finish with some theoretical issues concerning the possibility of harmonisation at transnational level.

Consent

Consent has been at the heart of many debates on the ethics of biobanking. It has come to be recognised that the notion of specific informed consent is problematic in relation to samples being collected for long term storage and other options, such as broad consent or dynamic consent (in an ongoing relationship with the donors), have been proposed. The basic principle at stake here is that autonomy will require the giving of informed consent for tissue samples to be taken where this involves a risk of direct harm to the sample donor. In relation to samples, the harm at issue is typically related to information associated with or derivable from the sample rather than to the physical intervention of taking the sample. There are also, however, questions about the extent to which the donor should have some say over the use of the samples after they have left the body – for example, whether they should be used for research x or research y. This is at the centre of the broad versus narrow consent debate. Over and above the differences in research context which affect appropriate consent, different understandings of what is required for consent and different cultural traditions affect what are perceived as the acceptable bounds of medical research. This is true even within Europe (Gaskell, 2010), but guidelines developed for initiatives such as Human Heredity and Health in Africa (www.h3Africa.org) have also recognised that consent is highly contextual.

From a point of view that wishes to maximise the value of samples, whichever ethical tradition is appealed to, consent needs to be sufficiently broad (Hansson et al., 2006; Helgesson, 2012; Peto et al., 2004). There remains, however, strong support for the view that consent needs to be specific, which may involve practical difficulties of reconsenting as new possibilities arise.

Data Protection: The Issues

As already mentioned, the potential harm that may accrue to a sample donor is primarily associated with the information associated with or derivable from a sample. There is an increasing awareness of the impossibility, in principle, of maintaining total privacy of data. Even though in practice new techniques of anonymisation and 'privacy by design' may make it very difficult to access personal data in research biobanking, it has been shown that it is not possible to guarantee privacy completely (Gymrek et al., 2013). It has been argued for some time that it is misleading to offer participants privacy protection in exchange for consent (Lunshof et al., 2008). The issues of privacy and consent are closely connected – and 'open' consent has been proposed, which, based on the principle of veracity, would make it clear to participants that their privacy cannot be guaranteed. Nevertheless, that does not relieve biobankers of their responsibilities to try to protect the data they have.

These issues arise within borders, but where samples and/or data move, additional concerns may arise. There are always technical risks associated with moving data and samples, as well as with ensuring secure storage once they have left one's control. Furthermore, the privacy protections in one jurisdiction may not apply in another, or if they do, their implementation may not be as precise. This second type of risk is especially difficult, as it may not be possible to overcome it with purely technical solutions and will demand mutual trust and understanding of values. Therefore, in transferring samples, an institution may be exposing donors to risks of what they might see as an abuse of their information.

Sharing the Benefits of Biomedical Research

An issue which potentially leads to the greatest acrimony concerns the sharing of benefits, especially where samples are collected in one country and transported to another and where there may be disparities in economic development, education or medical resources between the donor and recipient countries. It is important to establish systems to ensure that the obligation not to cause harm to research participants is observed but equally it may be necessary to consider whether some of the benefits arising out of research ought to be shared with the participants.

Outside of human tissue, the international Convention on Biological Diversity sets out the duties of benefit sharing from research carried out on indigenous plant and animal species, but it is inappropriate to extend this to human tissue research because of the (at least symbolic) status of the human genome as the common inheritance of all humanity (HUGO Ethics Committee, 2000; Schroeder and Lasén-Díaz, 2006).

A number of factors may be relevant in considering an appropriate benefit sharing regime. The donors of the samples in question clearly have to be considered whether the samples are collected specifically for transfer to another country or the decision to transfer them is made post collection. There are also issues concerning the local and international research teams (Choksi, et al., 2006). Last but not least, broader communities within the donor states ought to be taken into account.

Relatively early in the debate, the Human Genome Organisation's (HUGO) Ethical Legal and Social Issues (ELSI) Committee's *Statement on the Principled Conduct of Genetic Research* (1996) warned of the ethical dangers attached to offering rewards to individuals for donating samples (and recommended prohibition of the procurement of consent by individual inducement), but clearly distinguished benefits which are not likely to place undue pressure on tissue donors envisaging other benefits, such as 'technology transfer, local training, joint ventures, provision of health care or of information infrastructures, reimbursement of costs, or the possible use of a percentage of any royalties for humanitarian purposes'. The committee expanded on this in the context of international genomics research in its *Statement on Benefit Sharing* (HUGO, 2000). In that statement, the committee identified some key principles in the context of benefit sharing, notably solidarity and justice.

The HUGO Ethics Committee made a number of recommendations, the aggregate effect of which is to encourage a shift away from individual compensation without removing the possibility of community compensation (see Figure 2.1). In many cases, it may be the case that the donors are just a representative sample of the population or a section of the population. Ensuring that this wider community benefits from the results of any research will help to compensate this community for the use of 'their' genome. It is possible to re-think further the way in which biobanks are constructed and operated to fit more broadly with a solidarity approach, as in the 2011 report of the Nuffield Council on Bioethics, whereby the aim of the biobank would be primarily for the assistance of others, prioritising health needs over the generation of surplus value (Prainsack and Buyx, 2011). This report also raises the issue of the possibility of global solidarity and its potential impact on distribution of resources.

In regard to international sample collection, issues of cultural differences and different degrees of economic development may require special consideration as donors may be socially vulnerable (Garrafa, 2011). It is necessary to consider the relative states of development of all countries concerned in a transfer of biosamples, in relation to a number of aspects of justice. In particular, procedural justice: ensuring a just procedure by which the benefits of research are distributed

Recommendations:

1) that all humanity share in, and have access to, the benefits of genetic research.

2) that benefits not be limited to those individuals who participated in such research.

3) that there be prior discussion with groups or communities on the issue of benefit-sharing.

4) that even in the absence of profits, immediate health benefits as determined by community needs could be provided.

5) that at a minimum, all research participants should receive information about general research outcomes and an indication of appreciation.

6) that profit-making entities dedicate a percentage (e.g. 1% - 3%) of their annual net profit to healthcare infrastructure and/or to humanitarian efforts.

Figure 2.1   Statement on benefit sharing
Source: HUGO, 2000.

may be of great importance where there are any concerns about the abuse of a power imbalance by researchers from more developed countries. Procedures must be adequate to ensure that benefits are shared fairly with the donor communities.

Distributive justice also demands that all parties enjoy equitable access to the products of research; this may be of special relevance when the research is likely to lead to treatments which would ordinarily be out of reach of the donor community by reason of cost or scarcity. Garrafa (2011, p. 34) identifies two conditions for research to be considered cooperative and beneficial for developing countries:

(1) The research should seek therapeutic, preventative or diagnostic methods relating to the resolution of health problems that are a priority for the populations of the participating countries; and (2) ... accomplishing the research should enable technology transfer and development of skills of advanced investigative practices that can contribute towards achieving independence for the country regarding knowledge production.

Traditionally, international cooperation between research teams has been organised by way of bilateral agreements, which set out the degree of contribution of each party and how the benefits arising out of the research are to be split between them. Beyond that, however, there are the options of regulation and of harmonisation in ethics. Below we will explore each of these solutions in turn: we argue that they are not necessarily mutually exclusive.

Solutions?

Given all the issues outlined above, the question arises as to how to deal with them. In the previous paragraph bilateral agreements were mentioned, and we will examine a case study relating to this approach before exploring regulatory options and the complementary approach of harmonisation in ethics.

The Contractual Approach: The EUCoop Project

The 'Legal basis of EU-wide collaborations between biomaterial banks' or BMB-EUCoop project (BMB-EUCoop, 2013) aimed to examine, starting from the German perspective, many of the legal and ethical challenges which are faced by international biobanking collaborations (Goebel et al., 2010). The number of countries involved here was limited (UK, Netherlands, Austria and Switzerland are those examined from the German perspective). The project was set up primarily to address three major questions:

1. To what extent do foreign laws affect the property rights, personal rights and the right of informational self-determination of German biobanking donors?
2. To what extent does the transfer of biomaterials and data to foreign partners affect the property rights and the rights of commercial exploitation of German biobanks?
3. How can the positions of German biobanks and their donors be protected against the risks identified under 1 and 2, and how can such protection be enforced in practice, if so required?

The focus here is clear: how can the interests of the 'home' sample donors be protected in a transfer to other jurisdictions? The issues are partly legal and partly ethical, and it is not always easy to make a strict dichotomy between ethics and law. Several areas of potential conflict between the legal and ethical practices of different states were identified by the project as requiring explicit examination, these included: human and personal rights, property rights, medical professional regulations, commercialisation and intellectual property rights, supranational and international rights, benefit sharing, criminal law and prosecution and data and privacy protection.

A preliminary question for the study was the degree to which both ethical and legal standardisation had been established between the different countries involved: the varying results were revealed across the different areas of inquiry. In relation to both the personality and property rights of donors a good degree of legal and ethical convergence seemed to be present: similar requirements for protection of personality rights were identified in all five legal systems and the legal situation relating to property rights was found to be almost identical. This is perhaps not surprising, as these are the areas of ethics and law concerning which there is arguably the greatest agreement, at least within Europe. Whilst some minor differences in regulatory frameworks were found, it was suggested that any potentially negative consequences of divergent regulations could be remedied by appropriate stipulations in contractual agreements between parties in different states. This implied an implicit dependence upon ongoing negotiation. In relation to criminal law it was found that the legal frameworks across all five countries were fairly similar (complexities in the technical functioning of national and international criminal and depositive law were, however, seen to present particular obstacles) and the statutory requirement of physician confidentiality also applied to all research on human biomaterial in all of the countries covered by the study.

More problematic seemed to be those areas in which standardisation may be present, but where there is a significant degree of divergence in *implementation*. EU-wide standards have been outlined for the governance of the patenting of biomaterials under the EU Biopatenting Directive (Directive 98/44/EC); it was found, however, that significant differences exist between national approaches to the process of implementation. Similarly, in relation to data and privacy protection, a high degree of legal standardisation across different national jurisdictions had been achieved as a result of there having been a robust process resulting from the implementation of the EU Data Protection Directive (Directive 95/46/EC) – which still governs this area of practice at the time of writing. It was explicitly acknowledged, however, that inconsistencies in legal practice existed between different states, and that different levels of administrative stringency and efficiency in one country threatened to undermine standards in another.

Considerable differences were found to exist between different national medical professional regulations applicable to the international transfer of biomaterials (concerning storage, documentation and the requirement to inform donors of relevant research results). It was also found that international regulations governing biobanking practice often failed to provide clear-cut differences between normative and ethical regulations, or between 'soft' (not legally binding) law and nationally enforceable 'hard' law. This was seen to be particularly relevant to the issue of benefit-sharing: it was found that in this case, although most regulations are part of soft law and therefore not legally binding, researchers may still be subject to morally binding ethical obligations. The problems associated with this lack of basic standardisation tend to be negotiated by producing explicit contractual agreements which aim to protect the interests of internationally operating biobanks and their donors: this is a complex and challenging process that is likely to have significant practical impact on all collaborations.

Goebel et al. (2010) concluded that the best way to address the problematic issues which arise as biobanks from countries with substantially different legal and ethical systems collaborate is to ensure that detailed *contractual agreements* are made which cover the obligations and entitlements of all parties. This requires a process of ongoing negotiation between a diverse range of stakeholders. In a practical effort to help alleviate some of the problems found to be associated with a lack of standardisation and/or harmonisation in European biobanking, the BMB-EUCoop project produced a series of generic *texts* which were designed to address the issues outlined above and protect the interests of German biobanks and their donors: these included information for potential donors, consent forms and a contract for collaboration between German biobanks and international partners. These texts were explicitly designed so that they could be adapted to individual situations with minimal effort. This project, then, offers an example of how standards can be set and agreements made within a project but clearly as a more general solution it has limitations. We will now turn to external regulation.

External Regulation

The EU has sought to set common standards for how personal data is protected, to allow for free transfer of data between member states: it is recognised that flow of data is important. As indicated above, the time of writing data protection law in the EU is governed by the Data Protection Directive (Directive 95/46/EC). Although this system has had some success in creating a common regulatory regime for personal data in Europe, both an explosion in social media and changes in technology have led to a rapid increase in the amount of cross-border data movement and the complexity of data processing. These changes have exposed country-to-country differences in how the system works across the EU (Zita, 2010), and have put pressure on a regulatory regime that was designed in a different technological context.

As a Directive, the current regime had to be transposed into national law by member states in order to be effective against non-state actors. Additionally, under the current system data controllers have to do business with regulators in each country in which they operate. This lack of consistency both in terms of law and enforcement has been cited as one major reason for changes intended to create a level playing field across the EU (European Commission, 2010). In the context of biobanks, Budin-Ljøsne et al. (2012) have argued that the current legal framework supporting biobanking is focused at a national level to the detriment of international cooperation in the area.

It was proposed that the new regime (European Commission, 2012), which has been the object of intense scrutiny, discussion and amendment, would take the form of a regulation so that it would come into force without the need for transposition by member states: thus the same law would apply across the

EU. Genetic data are expressly recognised as an important category of personal information in the draft regulation, but the implications for biobankers who collect and store DNA samples have been difficult to clarify in the light of debate about removing a potential research exemption. Serious concerns have been expressed about the implications for biomedical research (Moraia et al., p. 3,013).

In terms of enforcement, national regulators will have greater obligations to cooperate with their counterparts in other member states and with the EU Commission, and data controllers will have one point of contact with regulators, with one regulator taking the lead in cross border cases (De Hert and Papakonstantinou, 2012).

The approach within the EU then has moved away from the significant autonomy granted to local regulators in order to provide uniformity. Although as Stephens et al. (2011) have argued, regulatory convergence in this area requires at least some level of social convergence, the trade-off between local autonomy and uniformity may be possible within the EU, where cultural differences – although present – are relatively surmountable. For transfers of data outside the EU, a different approach has been deemed necessary. Cultural differences may mean that the regulatory protections relating to personal data in other jurisdictions would be at odds with European values and principles, and could even be used to circumvent strict European rules governing data usage (Weber, 2013). Under the proposed regulation, transfers of personal data to countries outside the EU or to international organisations are restricted. A country, territory or processing sector may be approved generally by the Commission where it provides an adequate level of protection for personal data. In the absence of a decision from the Commission, data may be transferred subject to binding contractual or corporate rules being in force to protect the data. Where neither is possible, data transfer to a non-EU country would still be possible in a small number of circumstances, including where the data subject consents to the transfer in full knowledge of the risks involved. In setting out these safeguards, the proposed regulation is sensitive to differing cultural norms and allows the Commission to take a wide range of considerations into account in making its decision. Following the Edward Snowden affair, however, the proposals regarding international transfer of data, for example, to the United States, have been further strengthened (Traynor, 2013).

The need for the proposed regulation arises in the context of big data; a world where even the most apparently innocuous data may reveal deep insights into individuals' personal lives (Greengard, 2012). Similar problems have been shown to exist with anonymized biodata (Gymrek et al., 2013). This has led to a preference in the draft regulation for specific consent. Although some risks are present, however, there are good reasons why in some cases obtaining narrow consent from data subjects might not be desirable or possible in the context of biobanking. Unlike in other sectors, biobanks have traditionally had strong internal protections for personal data, with institutional review boards being specifically tasked to ensure that researchers maintain sound ethical practices in dealing with personal data. This ought to be considered by regulators in enacting data protection laws, and was provided for in the research exemption included in the Commission's original draft regulation.

In sum, the regulatory solution may produce harmonisation at the expense of flexibility, placing barriers in the way of research, especially international research.

The Possibilities of Harmonisation in Ethics

An approach which we see as complementary, rather than alternative, to the above is to seek harmonisation in ethics and values (Chadwick and Strange, 2009). When we turn from regulation to ethics, there may also be barriers to meaningful collaboration – for example, if completely different norms operate in different contexts about what people have consented to it may not be possible to compare results from one context to another. To a certain extent this is addressed by harmonisation in law, regulation and governance; for example, in the EU context, as discussed above. There are ethical issues outside the remit of law, hence the search for ethical standards. There is a question, however, over what would count as a standard in ethics, or whether harmonisation is the concept of choice: is there an ethical equivalent of the USB stick?

In 2009 Chadwick and Strange took inspiration from a musical analogy:

> It seems natural and right that music which is ... harmonious, should be highly regarded in civilised societies ... there is a clear correspondence between the concept of society as a mutually supportive commonwealth, and those manifestations of concert and theatre music which attract the collective approbation 'civilized'. ... Collective performance, as in singing the same text to different but interdependent vocal lines, can be regarded as the musical correlate of civilised democracy (Whittall, 2002, p. x).

It was this idea of different voices singing the same text to different vocal lines that seemed to hold an important insight – that harmonisation in ethics is best understood as a process, and not as an end point. Standards, or 'texts', can be produced for example in ethical guidelines (and in projects such as the EUCoop project), but the process of harmonisation in relation to these texts is something different. There may be, and indeed is, variation in interpretation of guidelines (which may of course occur in relation to law too, but we are not addressing that here) – the important question is, what is the acceptable scope for variation in relation to the text?

That there must be some limits to variation is clear: although in ethics agreement is not readily to be found on some issues, morality has a certain core. This gives a clue as to a potential response to possible criticism of the musical analogy, namely how one deals with those who are completely out of tune, or tone deaf. This raises deeper issues relating to the problem of the failure to accept moral reasoning at all, which we will not address here.

When we turn to the 'text' or standard, in this context a standard is a rule established to have action-guiding force. In the 2009 article we proceeded to identify three potential areas for standard setting in dealing with cross-border flow of data and materials: consent, feedback and privacy. We argued that the stronger the interests being protected, the more likely it was that a common standard would be required (and in fact this was found to be actualised in the EUCoop project). Likewise, room for different voices, variation in relation to the standard or text, would depend on the strength of those interests (how close they are to the 'core' of morality). From considering these three cases, we argued: that the strongest argument for a common standard existed in relation to informed consent (that is, an argument for some common standard; not *necessarily* for any particular form of informed consent, although in the context of biobanking, including across borders, consent needs to be sufficiently broad so that the purpose of the research can be achieved); there was room for variation in relation to feedback, depending on local conditions; and, as regards privacy, the thinking in this area is in a phase of rapid development and we can no longer assume that protection can be guaranteed (cf. Lunshof et al., 2008; Gymrek et al., 2013). The ethical considerations here are clearly intertwined with political considerations, including global ones, as can be seen from the impact of international concerns about data which go far beyond the issues relevant to biobanking, but which inevitably have an impact upon them. It is important in these circumstances to return to the ethical issues at stake and the important interests of individuals and communities which may be disadvantaged as a side effect of global politics.

Conclusion

We have examined some areas of concern with regard to transfer of samples across borders, consent, data protection and benefit sharing, and three different approaches to dealing with them, contractual agreements, regulation and ethical harmonisation. Each has their advantages and drawbacks, but we suggest that the ethical harmonisation project should be regarded as complementary, and not an alternative, to the contractual and regulatory approaches, otherwise the voices of researchers and research participants – and ultimately patients – may be overshadowed by the louder tunes of law and regulation.

References

BMB-EUCoop, 2013. *Legal basis of EU-wide biobanking cooperation.* [online] Available at: <http://www.tmfev.de/EnglishSite/Topics/Biobanking andmolecularmedicine/V01002BMBEUCoopEN.aspx> [Accessed 8 July 2013].

Budin-Ljøsne, I., Harris, J.R., Kaye, J., Knoppers, B.M. and Tassé, A.M., 2012. ELSI Challenges and strAtegies of National Biobank Infrastructures. *Norsk Epidemiologi*, 21(2), pp. 155–60.

Chadwick, R. and Strange, H., 2009. Harmonisation and Standardisation in Ethics and Governance: Conceptual and practical challenges. In: H. Widdows and C. Mullen, eds. 2009. *The Governance of Genetic Information: Who decides.* Cambridge: Cambridge University Press, pp. 201–13.

Chen, H. and Gottweis, H., 2013. Stem Cell Treatments in China: Rethinking the patient role in the global bio-economy. *Bioethics*, 27(4), pp. 194–207.

Choksi, D.A., Parker, M. and Kwiatkowski, D.P., 2006. Data Sharing and Intellectual Property in a Genomic Epidemiology Network: Policies for large-scale research collaboration. *Bulletin of the World Health Organization*, 84, pp. 382–7.

De Hert, P. and Papakonstantinou, V., 2012. The Proposed Data Protection Regulation Replacing Directive 95/46/EC: A sound system for the protection of individuals. *Computer Law and Security Review*, 28(2), pp. 130–42.

European Commission, 1995. *Data Protection Directive.* Directive 95/46/ EC. [online] Available at: <http://eur-lex.europa.eu/LexUriServ/LexUriServ. do?uri=CELEX:31995L0046:en:HTML> [Accessed 22 December 2013].

———, 1998. *EU Biopatenting Directive.* Directive 98/44/EC. [online] Available at: <http://eurlex.europa.eu/smartapi/cgi/sga_doc?smartapi!celexapi!prod!CE LEXnumdoc&lg=en&numdoc=31998L0044&model=guichett> [Accessed 22 December 2013].

———, 2010. A Comprehensive Approach on Personal Data Protection in the European Union. *Communication from the Commission to the European Parliament, the Council, the Economic and Social Committee and the Committee of the Regions* (COM, 609). [online] Available at: <http://ec.europa. eu/justice/news/consulting_public/0006/com_2010_609_en.pdf> [Accessed 22 December 2013].

———, 2012. *Proposal for the EU general data protection regulation,* [online] Available at: <http://ec.europa.eu/justice/data-protection/document/review 2012/com_2012_11_en.pdf> [Accessed 8 July 2013].

Garrafa, V., 2011. International Research. In: R. Chadwick, H. ten Have and E.M. Meslin, eds. *The SAGE Handbook of Health Care Ethics.* London: SAGE, p. 342.

Gaskell, G., Stares, S., Allansdottir, A., Allum, N., Castro, P. et al., 2010. *Europeans and Biotechnology in 2010 Winds of Change?* Available through: University of Essex repository <http://repository.essex.ac.uk/2291/> [Accessed 22 December 2013].

Goebel, J.W., Pickardt, T., Bedau, M., Fuchs, M., Lenk, C. et al., 2010. Legal and Ethical Consequences of International Biobanking from a National Perspective: The German BMB-EUCoop project. *European Journal of Human Genetics*, 18(5), pp. 522–5.

Greengard, S., 2012. Advertising Gets Personal. *Commununications of the ACM*, 55(8), pp. 18–20.

Gymrek, M., McGuire, A.L., Golan, D., Halperin, E. and Erlich, Y., 2013. Identifying Personal Genomes by Surname Inference. *Science*, 339(6,117), pp. 321–4.

Hansson, M.G., Dillner, J., Bartram, C.R., Carlson, J.A. and Helgesson, G., 2006. Should Donors be Allowed to Give Broad Consent to Future Biobank Research? *The Lancet Oncology*, 7(3), pp. 266–9.

Helgesson, G., 2012. In Defense of Broad Consent. *Cambridge Quarterly of Healthcare Ethics*, 21(01), pp. 40–50.

HUGO ELSI Committee, 1996. *Statement on the Principled Conduct of Genetics Research*. Human Genome Organisation. [online] Available at: <http://www1. umn.edu/humanrts/instree/geneticsresearch.html> [Accessed 12 June 2013].

HUGO Ethics Committee, 2000. *Statement on Benefit Sharing*. Human Genome Organisation. [online]. Available at: http://www.hugo-international.org/img/ benefit_sharing_2000.pdf [Accessed 13 June 2013].

Lunshof, J.E., Chadwick, R., Vorhaus, D.B. and Church, G.M., 2008. From Genetic Privacy to Open Consent. *Nature Reviews Genetics*, 9(5), pp. 406–11.

Moraia, L.B., Kaye, J. and Griffin, H., 2013. The Implications of the Proposed EU Data Protection Reform on Biomedical Research. *Bionews*, 12 August. [online] Available at: <www.bionews.org.uk> [Accessed 9 December 2013].

Peto, J., Fletcher, O. and Gilham, C., 2004. Data Protection, Informed Consent, and Research: Medical research suffers because of pointless obstacles. *BMJ: British Medical Journal*, 328(7,447), p. 1,029.

Prainsack, B. and Buyx, A., 2011. *Solidarity: Reflections on an emerging concept in bioethics*. London: Nuffield Council on Bioethics.

Salter, B., 2008. Governing Stem Cell Science in China and India: Emerging economies and the global politics of innovation. *New Genetics and Society*, 27(2), pp. 145–59.

Salter, B. and Salter, C., 2007. Bioethics and the Global Moral Economy: The cultural politics of human embryonic stem cell science. *Science, Technology & Human Values*, 32(5), pp. 554–81.

Schroeder, D. and Lasén-Díaz, C., 2006. Sharing the Benefits of Genetic Resources: From biodiversity to human genetics. *Developing World Bioethics*, 6(3), pp. 135–43.

Stephens, N., Atkinson, P. and Glasner, P., 2011. Internationaliser des standards, mettre en banque avec confiance. *Revue d'anthropologie des connaissances*, 5(2), pp. 260–86.

Traynor, I., 2013. New EU Rules to Curb Transfer of Data to US After Edward Snowden Revelations. *The Guardian*, 17 October. [online] Available at: <www. theguardian.com> [Accessed 15 November 2013].

Weber, R.H., 2013. Transborder Data Transfers: Concepts, regulatory approaches and new legislative initiatives. *International Data Privacy Law*, 3(2), pp. 117–30.

Whittall, A., 2002. Harmony. In: A. Latham, ed. *Oxford Companion to Music*. Oxford: Oxford University Press, p. 561.

Zika, E., Paci, D., Braun, A., RijKers-Defrasne, S., Deschênes, M. et al., 2010. *Biobanks in Europe: Prospects for harmonisation and networking*. Institute for Prospective and Technological Studies, Joint Research Centre. [online] Available at: http://ideas.repec.org/p/ipt/iptwpa/jrc57831.html [Accessed 8 July 2013].

Chapter 3

Masculinity Under the Knife: Filipino Men, Trafficking and the Black Organ Market in Manila, the Philippines[1]

Sallie Yea

Introduction

Recent social science scholarship on the global organ trade has highlighted the importance of considering the social, cultural, moral/religious and economic milieu in which organs are commercially received (Crowley-Matoka and Lock, 2006; Hamdy, 2010; Kierans, 2011; Parry, 2008; Sanal, 2011; Shimazono, 2008) and, to a lesser extent, provided (Scheper-Hughes, 2008, 2011). These accounts suggest that universal notions of commodification and exploitation, such as those put forward in media accounts and in studies such as Carney's (2011) global survey of the organ trade and in some of Scheper-Hughes' early work on the kidney trade (2000, 2003), be tempered in favour of a view of these processes as representing 'unstable commodification' involving, 'forms that embody the equivocal relationship that communities and individuals have to the concept and practice of bodily commodification' (Parry, 2008, p. 1,139). Using these strands of inquiry as a starting point, in this chapter I explore the meanings of commercial kidney provision amongst male providers drawn from the Manila slum of Baseco. This area of Manila has achieved notoriety as a 'hotspot' for organ trafficking in the Philippines and has predominantly been characterised as an 'organ bazaar' in which poor men are exploited and trafficked in a global market for cheap kidneys. This framing however obfuscates, 'how transplantation becomes a site for the enactment of social processes and relationships, particularly those adversely affecting women, children and the lives of the poor, both within and across borders' (Kierans, 2011, p. 1,473).

In taking socio-cultural processes, relationships and situated meanings as my starting point for discussion, the chapter has two aims relating specifically to the gendered meanings men ascribe to selling a kidney. First, one of the most striking characteristics of these providers is that, at least amongst cases documented, the vast majority are economically marginal men. In the Philippines I inquired

---

1   This chapter was first published in *Gender, Place & Culture: A Journal of Feminist Geography*, 7 October 2013. Copyright © 2013 Routledge.

to key informants in Baseco and during non-governmental organisation (NGO) interviews about the prevalence of female providers and was told that there were 'some women' who sold a kidney but they were outnumbered by about 100:1 by men.[2] This raises interesting questions about the ways poor men invoke local inscriptions of Filipino masculinity through processes of bodily commodification associated with commercial kidney provision. In broad discussions of organ trafficking, the links between constructions and performances of masculinity for economically and socially marginal men and commercial organ provision may be missed in accounts only focusing on men's exploitation without attending to the complex ways exploitation and marginalisation may be intertwined with gendered idioms.

The second and related aim of the chapter is to explore the ways men manoeuvre and critique discourses of exploitation that situate them as victims of trafficking. There has been a significant amount of critical scholarship on representations and discourses in human trafficking that promote trafficked persons as 'spectacle' (Andrijasevic, 2007) drawing on what prominent feminist lawyer Ratna Kapur (2002) dubs 'the tragedy of the victim rhetoric' (see also Doezema, 2010; Hua and Nigorizawa, 2010; Lainez, 2010; Pajnik, 2010). One of the key suggestions of this scholarship is that the victim rhetoric obscures trafficked persons agency, casting them as powerless, duped innocents lacking the ability to manage or overcome their situations of exploitation. Whilst these arguments have been made largely in relation to women in the sex industry, as Rebecca Surtees (2008) also notes, men can be particularly 'unwilling victims' under these rhetorical mores. Following this, the second aim of the chapter is to explore questions about representations of trafficking and exploitation for the men in this study and the subsequent invocation of Filipino masculinity involving heroism. In relation to this second aim, I ask: how do men attempt to contest victim discourses and simultaneously assert their own critique of their positioning within the organ market through local inscriptions of masculinity?

Through discussion of these two interrelated issues regarding the interstices between organ trafficking, masculinity and economic marginality I wish to contribute to recent discussions in geography and related disciplines concerning masculinity, particularly as it expressed amongst non-Western, economically and socially marginal men. Critical geographers have made important contributions to discussions of masculinity and contemporary processes, such as migration (Datta et al., 2009; Herbert, 2008; May et al., 2008), ethnicity (Hopkins, 2006, 2007), labour geographies (McDowell, 2003) and material culture and representations

---

2   All participants were asked about the approximate total number of commercial kidney providers in Baseco and about the gender breakdown of this total. Responses were remarkably uniform with men stating that only a few women had sold a kidney and there were far more men who engaged in the practice. NGOs working on this issue can only suggest the gender distribution of participants and their assessments tended to confirm those of the participants.

(Jackson et al., 1999). However, the vast majority of these discussions have focused on Western, particularly British, contexts, even where they are concerned with non-White/minority ethnicities. To a certain extent Robyn Longhurst's (2000, p. 443) summation there 'are still many areas within the discipline of geography where discussions of masculinity are notably absent' remains a truism particularly for development geographies. Certainly engagements with human trafficking generally and organ sales in particular, as well as Asian contexts have been lacking in such emerging sub-disciplinary engagements with masculinity.

Before turning to my analysis in the chapter a brief discussion of ethics, methodology and the field site is warranted. I then describe the ways organ sales and transplantations are organised for the men in this study. Academic discussions of masculinity and socio-economic marginality tend to have as a central focus the ways alternative or 'resistant' masculinities articulate with hegemonic masculinity and the expressive forums and forms they adopt. The third part of the chapter therefore briefly reviews these discussions and problematises the assumption of much of this literature that non-hegemonic masculinity is occupied by men without significant social power and economic resources, and vice versa. I suggest here that this binary is overly simplistic and in reality my participants' imaginings of a successful man involve a complex interplay of hegemonic ideals. In the main part of the chapter I discuss the ways Filipino masculinity intersects with commercial organ provision producing a new constellation through which masculinity is (re)configured. This discussion is divided into two parts: the first focusing on men's gendered roles as breadwinners and within the family; the second focusing on the ways heroism is invoked in relation to kidney selling. In concluding, I reflect on the insights gained from discussion in the chapter for understandings of the interstices between masculinity and exploitative kidney sales where Filipino men are concerned.

Methodology, Ethics and the Field

The chapter is based on the first phase of a qualitative study of commercial kidney providers in Manila conducted in 2009 and 2011. Fifteen men participated in in-depth semi-structured interviews in 2009, which were conducted in the home of a key informant in the squatter area of Baseco, where the men also lived. As well as these interviews follow up fieldwork was conducted in 2011 in which I sought out the original participants and visited their homes and assessed their family, relational and financial circumstances through follow up semi-structured interviews. Several topics were discussed during these interviews, including the men's family and educational backgrounds, lives and work in Baseco, motivations for selling a kidney and the subsequent recruitment process, details of hospitalisation and transplantation, and life in the short to medium term post-transplantation. In the follow up fieldwork all but one of the original participants was re-interviewed. During the second fieldwork phase non-formal interactions and observations were also undertaken, particularly relating to bodily performances in Baseco.

A qualitative approach to the research was adopted because I was particularly interested in ways men interpreted, reconstructed and performed their experiences of commercial kidney provision, particularly men's moral, social and gendered framing of this. Telling their story on their own terms was also important in enabling men to realise some degree of authorship over their experience and whilst I would stop well short of attempting to pose this as empowering for these men, they were nonetheless able to claim some degree of control over their narratives which arguably has been lost in broad accounts of their trafficking experiences.

Difficulties associated with researching 'hidden populations' of trafficked persons have been widely noted (Brennan, 2005) and include access and building rapport with 'victims'. Access to this population was also difficult insofar as commercial kidney providers in Manila are not currently supported as 'victims of trafficking' meaning that access through shelters or other support processes is irrelevant. Men who participated in this study were accessed through a personal contact (my Uncle) who resides in Baesco, which is the largest slum settlement in Manila and the most infamous source district for commercial organ providers in the Manila capital region. Unlike trafficking in other sectors where internal or transnational migration is involved, and where populations may be highly mobile (especially if they are in migration destinations, shelters or transit areas) kidney providers returned home to Baseco after their transplantation and have continued to reside there, at least during the term of the research thus far.

Access to vulnerable and erstwhile trafficked populations does not necessarily guarantee good research outcomes. Trust and rapport are important for disclosure of often traumatic, shameful and distressing experiences. Because my husband is Filipino and has relatives living in the field site, his role as research assistant was pivotal in achieving trust amongst the men we interviewed. Oakley (1981) and Scheyvens and Leslie (2000) suggest the importance of shared gender in achieving disclosure, particularly with participants who may be oppressed and/or who are asked to discuss intimate, emotionally sensitive or traumatic experiences. In addition, the existence of a male relative co-resident in Baseco worked to overcome possible class differentials between participants and the researcher and her assistant, so whilst there were clear power asymmetries between the researcher and participants, there were also important sites of accord.

Apart from issues of access, trust and rapport trafficking research can present heightened ethical concerns, including fear of retribution from traffickers, re-traumatisation through re-telling their experiences, insecurities in migration status (especially where the victim is still residing in the trafficking destination country), and immediate needs generated by physical/health and economic problems. But most of these concerns have been identified through research with women and girls trafficked into the sex industry (for example, WHO, 2003). Little has been written about issues of access and ethics where researching organ trafficking is concerned (though see Scheper-Hughes, 2004). Some of the broad issues parallel those of trafficking in other sectors, particularly relating to the vulnerabilities trafficked persons can face upon exiting their situations of exploitation. But the specific ethical issues in conducting research with the men in the study derived principally from only two of these concerns, namely their diminished health and economic positions post-transplantation. Referrals to non-government organisations (NGOs) in Manila focusing on commercial organ provision were made for some participants where they requested this. Addressing problems of financial exploitation of participants was beyond the scope of the research since it required legal actions aimed at realising compensation, which in the Philippines is a lengthy process with no assurances of a positive outcome.

Organ Trafficking: Going Under the Knife in Manila

There are many different ways in which kidney sales are organised, both in Manila and elsewhere in the Philippines (Asia ACTS, n.d.; Gagaloc, 2008; Mendoza, 2010). The men who participated in this research fell predominantly into a cohort that sought out 'kidney brokers' themselves or were approached by a broker in their neighbourhood. For these men the modus operandi of commercial organ provision was defined by the broker charging a fee for facilitating the sale of the kidney. The broker's role is to connect the provider and a doctor that is willing to perform the transplant. The doctor, or sometimes other hospital staff, in turn connects with prospective renal failure patients abroad or, in some cases, in the Philippines itself. The broker receives a fee from all three parties involved in the transaction; the provider, the hospital (who pays the broker as a recruiter) and the patient. The broker plays a pivotal role in the organ trade in Manila and, arguably heightens the level of exploitation of the provider through the extraction of a hefty fee and creating vague and unfulfilled terms of agreement governing the transaction (Mendoza, 2010).

The men in this study described how their initial agreement to the sale was followed by one or two visits to the hospital for health screening and blood matching tests which would ensure their suitability as a provider and compatibility with the kidney recipient. For some men only a few days would pass before they were called to the hospital for their operation, whilst for others the wait extended for several weeks. After being admitted to the hospital men were usually operated the following day. Men described being anesthetised and knowing the impossibility of withdrawing at that point. Upon waking and despite severe pain, the men were normally confined for only one further day and then discharged after a single visit from the attending doctor who would give the men a large plastic bag of painkillers and bandages and advise them to come back for more prescriptions if they required them. Some of the men were told they could have one or several 'free check ups' if they wanted it, whilst others were not given a choice to avail follow-up health care. The men returned to Baseco to recuperate under the care of their families (who sometimes were oblivious to their husband's/son's/father's decisions until post-transplantation) and, in many cases, the care of other men who had sold a kidney previously.

Although the circumstances under which kidney transactions occur differ amongst providers in Baseco and Luzon more broadly – with some men having sought out a 'broker' to mediate the sale, and others having to be 'convinced' by a recruiter to sell a kidney – it is clear that the men who provide a kidney on Manila's commercial organ market are operating in a situation of 'imperfect knowledge' (Mendoza, 2010), with brokers and medical practitioners, as well as the transplant recipients, benefitting disproportionately from the transactions. It might well be argued that these men are trafficked, in the sense that their vulnerability as economically marginal family breadwinners is the key inducement to selling a kidney and they are undoubtedly exploited in the process (Yea, 2010). This view is in line with the definition of trafficking put forward in the United Nations Trafficking Protocol (2000), where trafficking is understood as:

> the recruitment, transportation, transfer, harbouring or receipt of persons, by means of the threat or use of force or other forms of coercion, of abduction, of fraud, of deception, of the abuse of power or of a position of vulnerability or of the giving or receiving of payments or benefits to achieve the consent of a person having control over another person, for the purpose of exploitation. Exploitation shall include, at a minimum, the exploitation of the prostitution of others or other forms of sexual exploitation, forced labour or services, slavery or practices similar to slavery, servitude or the removal of organs.

The Philippines own anti-trafficking law (RA 9208) (2003) is modelled on the UN Protocol.[3] For kidney sellers in Manila both the Protocol and RA 9208 are both relevant to their experiences insofar as it is their status as impoverished and poorly educated slum dwellers that leads to their vulnerability and subsequent exploitation in the kidney market. Further, men were universally deceived about both the financial and health consequences of these transactions. Indeed, responding to the accusation of organ trafficking in Luzon (Asia ACTS, n.d.), the Philippines government has recently regulated the practice of commercial organ provision and criminalised the organ trade utilising legal provisions contained in the Anti-Trafficking in Persons Act. Although this has dampened the market it has certainly not eliminated it, with commercial organ providers continuing to be exploited (personal communication, representative of Asia ACTs, May 2012; see also Bagayaua, 2009). These experiences of 'going under the knife' and trafficking categorisations tell us little however about the motives for providers to sell a kidney or the consequences of their involvement in this market and how this informs and

---

3   In 2003 the Republic Act (RA) 9208 came into force. It related to the trafficking of persons for a range of purposes, including commercial sexual exploitation, forced labour and organ trafficking. It defines organ trafficking (Section 4, paragraph G) as, 'To recruit, hire, adopt, transport or abduct a person by means of threat or use of force, fraud, deceit, coercion or intimidation for the purpose of removal or sale or organs of said person' (Republic of Philippines, 2003).

in turn reconfigures their sense of masculinity. Such an undertaking requires us to look beyond broad iterations of exploitative transactions to the narratives of the providers themselves.

Masculinity, Marginality and Globalisation: An Overview

Whilst literature in geography and related disciplines on gender, marginality and contemporary global processes and structures has burgeoned recently most discussions focus on women, particularly as they relate to the ways women are situated in and manoeuvre structures and relations of inequality (see, for example, Ehrenreich and Hochschild, 2004), including trafficking (Beeks and Amir, 2006). Women have also figured prominently in discussions of body-parts commodification, particularly regarding commercial surrogacy (Hochschild, 2009). Yet scholarship in geography and related disciplines on contemporary masculinity has focused less on the themes of exploitation and marginality and more on the avenues through which masculinity is expressed and reconfigured, particularly through migration, ethnicity/minority status, class and labour markets, and material culture and representations. Whilst contributing valuable insights, these foci do not necessarily attend to the ways exploitation, inequality and masculinity may be intertwined in many men's experiences, especially in the third world. Hung Cam Thai (2005, p. 316) points out that despite 'assertions of employing gender as a key analytical category in migratory and transnational processes ... there is virtually no focus on the meanings of masculinity in globalisation among ... men of colour'. What work has appeared on subaltern men and masculinity in the context of globalised relations has focused almost entirely on migration, particularly for low skilled work (Datta et al., 2009; Herbert, 2008; McKay, 2007; May et al., 2008; Osella and Osella, 2000; Pribilsky, 2012), including for the Philippines (McKay, 2010, 2011; Pingol, 2000).

Whilst migration has been an important forum in advancing understandings of globalisation and subaltern masculinity, trafficking and related forms of exploitation has also belatedly, albeit rather peripherally appeared within these discussions (Surtees, 2008). Rebecca Surtees (2011) study of East European men in the long haul fishing industry recognises the importance of trafficking's effects on men's sense of identity and selfhood, including the ways they experience and must manoeuvre failed migration projects in light of their family roles at home. Her research suggests that masculinity is compromised as a result of the experience of trafficking, something Sallie Yea also found in preliminary research with trafficked fishermen from the Philippines (Yea, 2014).[4] Research specifically on the kidney

---

4   Although academic research has not been particularly attentive to the topic of men as trafficked persons, some international NGO studies have provided interesting insights into the issue. A recent study of unsafe migration and reintegration of trafficked and exploited persons in three provinces in Cambodia, for example, found that men were more

trade has confirmed many of these findings about the dilution of men's familial and economic roles as providers. Drawing on Scheper-Hughes' work, Parry (2008) notes in relation to Moldova that, 'men who have sold a kidney to escape debt, are now being stigmatised as male "prostitutes" as they are no longer able to partake in the only labour available to men in their rural communities, heavy agricultural or construction work. They are being excommunicated from their orthodox eastern European churches, alienated from families and friends, and if single, excluded from marriage' (p. 1,142). But while these post-trafficking trajectories tell us much about how men's positions are diluted through the experience of trafficking, especially as they negotiate the shame of economic failure and bodily derogation, they hold few insights into the question of how men who sell their body parts construct their decisions or negotiate their failure drawing on a repertoire of tropes of masculinity.

Arguably, current discussions of masculinity in the social sciences are not particularly helpful in illuminating the answers to this question. A critical gaze over the extensive literature on contemporary masculinities alerts us to an important absence, namely non-hegemonic masculinities in non-Western, and specifically third world contexts. The recent literature on masculinities has been dominated by discussions of hegemonic masculinity as originally developed by Raewyn Connell (1995), who proposed that at any one time in any given society there will be an ideal way of being a successful man. Amongst the many who have subsequently proposed what these elements may include, Townsend (2002) has been influential in his description of hegemonic masculinity in the West as involving an (often elusive) combination of economic providership, homeownership, marriage and fatherhood. But, as noted by others, the idea of a hegemonic masculinity in any given social and cultural milieu can produce misleading binaries in which non-hegemonic masculinities are posed as alternative constructions (Demetriou, 2001). Will Courtenay (2000, p.1,391) suggests that, 'when men and boys are denied access to the social power and resources necessary for constructing hegemonic masculinity, they must seek other resources for constructing gender that validate their masculinity' (see also Messerschmidt, 1993). These resources include hyper-masculine practices associated with violence, crime and, sometimes, wounded bodies and suffering, particularly in prisons, the urban street gang or amongst soldiers (Connell, 1992; Courtenay, 1999; Courtenay and Sabo, 2001; Messner and Sabo, 1994). This literature assumes that lack of access to social power and political-economic resources will lead marginalised (read lower class men and ethnic and sexual minority men) to configure their masculinity in terms which depart from hegemonic masculinity. Because these suggestions have been made largely in relation to Western contexts, does not however necessarily mean they hold universal validity.

---

likely to be trafficked than women and that women were far more likely to be recognised as trafficked and receive support. Other studies have documented the widespread presence of trafficking in the long haul fishing industry in Asia; a sector almost exclusively involving male employees (for example, IOM, 2009; Yea, forthcoming).

Despite their socio-economic positions, male kidney sellers in Baseco draw on normative – rather than 'resistant' – ideas of what it means to be a successful man in the Philippines, particularly concerning heroism and family providership. In relation to lower class Filipino seafarers McKay (2011, p. 4) similarly found that, 'this group of workers, channelled into the lower ends of the global market and subordinated at work, nevertheless often construct themselves as "masculine exemplars" or idealised versions of masculinity'. Nonetheless, I refrain from celebrating commercial organ provision as an important locus for restoring these men's masculinity through global outlets, but argue that the experience of commercial organ provision under exploitative circumstances holds contradictory implications for men's sense of selfhood and their 'success' as men. It is to a consideration of these complicated negotiations around masculinity in Baseco that we now turn.

Masculinity Under the knife

Haligi ng Tahanan (Pillar of the Family)

Pingol's (2001, p. 7) in-depth treatment of contemporary Filipino masculinity is framed in the context of rapidly increasing outmigration of Filipino women for work abroad. She identifies, 'being good providers, virile sex partners, firm and strong fathers' as being at the centre of constructions of Filipino masculinity. It is these traits that render men *kinalalaki*, or worthy of respect from others. Filipino men are thought to be 'self-actualised' (*ganap nalalaki*) if they have started a family and can demonstrate that they are able to look after the family's welfare. This standard of masculinity is reflected in the expression *haligi ng tahanan* (literally, pillar of the family). When men become househusbands and perform 'mothering' and other domestic duties at home as their wives migrate for work, challenges to the constitution of masculinity are bound to emerge, leading men to attempt to reinterpret these elements of masculinity. Her arguments have been underscored by others writing on the social effect of Philippine labour migration (see, for example, Parrenas, 2008). This work (see also McKay, 2009) highlights a more general observation that the male breadwinner model remains a normative tenet of masculinity amongst Filipinos. Rubio and Green (2009) similarly found that Filipino masculinity differs markedly from Western ideals because of the emphasis on family orientation and less focus on aggression, emotional restriction, dominance and an over-emphasis on strength. Men's providership in the familial space is one of the most significant locus for masculinity in the Philippines and emerged often within men's narratives about their decisions to sell a kidney.

It is estimated that around 3,000 of Baseco's 100,000 residents have sold a kidney, with the vast majority being men (Aguilar and Siruno, 2004). Of the 15 men who participated in this research, 13 were married with children. Of the remaining two participants, one was gay and therefore unmarried (in the Philippines same sex marriage is prohibited by law) and the other was single at the time of the initial interview in 2009 (though had become married in the interim between the first and second field visits). All these men cited economic considerations as the major motive for selling a kidney, and we discussed at length the financial situation of the men prior to their transplantation, as well as the economic benefits anticipated. In this regard Ro's[5] narrative was a common one amongst the men:

> I earn PHP 180 a day and I am the only one who works in my family. Our cost for living for the day is about PHP120, so we live hand-to-mouth. Whatever is left we must try to save in case one of the children becomes sick or needs extra money at school.

However, delving more deeply into the men's motivations the economic imperatives that informed men's decisions were themselves embedded within the men's familial situations and perceived responsibilities. This was the case for the two single participants as well as those who were married, with the two single men giving all the money from the sale to their parents. Al said that he decided to sell a kidney because he had migrated from a poor rural area in provincial Luzon to Manila in order to find work and send money back to his parents who were struggling on their farm. He recounted:

> After the operation I was paid USD 2000 and I sent every single cent back to my parents. Since coming to Manila my work has been only casual and not enough for my own needs, let alone to send money back home. I didn't tell my parents what I was planning to do, but after I gave them the money I told them how I had earned it. They were really angry with me and upset, but they still accepted the money. I don't have much contact with them now … It makes me happy that I could keep my promise that I could support them.

Al's admission parallels those of many Filipino migrant workers who must negotiate the mismatch between anticipated and actual earnings. For overseas Filipino workers this can produce considerable shame (*hiya*) and scrutiny within the home community, but Al's experience shows that internal migrants are not immune to these cultural codes around shame and obligation either. The other single participant, Jo also gave all but a small proportion of the money from the kidney sale to his parents.

For the other men supporting marital families was the primary motive for selling a kidney. The men saw the money they would gain as contributing to the building of a proper house, supporting a small business, paying for the cost of children's education, or a combination of all these. Re said this:

> I have four kids and my wife. We don't live in a proper house and my work is only casual as a day labourer. Some days I get work and some days I don't …

---

5   Pseudonyms are used when referring to participants.

Well, the kids' school is free but I can't afford the extra costs, like for books and excursions and things. I don't want the kids to end up working like me. I don't want my wife and kids to live like this [in a tin shack] all their lives.

Re, like all the other participants except one performed manual labour in their work, and all these men were either day labourers, causal *cargadors* (carriers of goods from the docked cargo ships to the railway or road transport centre), fishermen (as Baseco is on tidal flats near the main port in Manila Bay), or tricycle drivers. Most earned between PP 50–200 per day (USD 1–4), if they worked at all.

Assuring the welfare of the family by investing the money from a kidney transplant in a small business venture was at the back of many of the men's minds (only two of the married participants did not plan to start a business with the money they would gain from the kidney sale). Je stated that he planned to start a small food stall (*carenderia*):

We have our house already. I wanted to extend at the front of the house with a food stall. I bought all the things we needed – like pots, pans and a stove – and we ran that stall for three years.

Many of the men who earned a living through fishing in small boats in Manila Bay desired to own a boat of their own; to rent a fishing vessel meant that half the day's catch had to be shared with the owner of the boat, which depleted these men's income considerably. Two participants did buy boats with their transplantation money, with another stating that he would have purchased a boat had he received all the money he was promised. Being able to purchase a boat meant moving from a hand-to-mouth existence to a position where funds could be reserved for children's needs and, participants were keen to emphasise, to prevent the wife or children having to work. This last point deserves further elaboration.

It was in men's narration of the possibility of their children or wives having to work that they touched on the male breadwinner role most explicitly and urgently. A few of the participants had been forced into financial situations where there was no option but for their wife or even children to work and men spoke repeatedly with shame that they were powerless to prevent this. Gi's disclosure was revealing in this regard:

We were so broke because my mother-in-law got sick and I had to give our small savings to her for treatment. At that point my wife decided to take work doing people's laundry. I was so ashamed that she was working and earning more than me. It's not that I minded her working if that's what she wanted to do; it was the fact that there was no choice and she had to do it because I couldn't support the family.

Re also recounted with obvious guilt that his oldest son had to drop out of high school at the age of 12 years and begin working selling newspapers in Baseco's large market:

> I have three boys and my oldest son dropped out of school so the other two could continue on with their studies. I am proud of him in a way, and I knew he did it [dropped out] so that I didn't have to pay the extra costs for school. But imagine yourself; how could you let your kid work because you can't make enough money to support your own family?

In both Gi's and Re's cases it was engagement of family members in work out of necessity that ultimately motivated them to seek out brokers to sell a kidney.

Despite these aspirations for family security, for various reasons the men's plans rarely came to fruition. Returning to Al's narrative, for example, giving all the kidney money to his parents left him back where he started in his attempts to fulfil his familial responsibilities. On the return research visit in 2011, we found Al already married and living in a two square metre shack with a dirt floor (see Figure 3.1). He was still fishing but on a vessel owned by someone else. He was not able to afford to buy his own boat nor, as he desired, to build a 'decent house' to start a family. Many of the other providers were tragically affected by natural disaster and lost the new houses and businesses that they had purchased with money from their kidney sales. Fires, which are commonplace within Manila's squatter areas, destroyed the new homes that seven of the participants had built, whilst cyclones had broken the boats of both the men that had made these purchases with their kidney money. The fires that destroyed the men's new houses also destroyed the businesses that they started. When we discussed these outcomes many of the men reflected that this was their 'punishment' for going against God and defiling the body He endowed them with. The only provider in the study who continued to benefit financially from his transplantation received an annual 'gift' from the recipient of his kidney (an overseas Filipino woman living in the United States), which totalled around two months of his income as a hairdresser. He considered himself lucky in light of the circumstances his *compadres* found themselves in; without a kidney and having lost the businesses that were to assure their financial futures.

The exploitation in the kidney sales, particularly the absence of follow up healthcare, is particularly relevant in light of these livelihood losses and has also been noted by Scheper-Hughes in relation to both men in the Philippines and Moldova (2011). Because the men in this study were unable (or unwilling) to avail basic short- and long-term post-operative medical care their health had diminished considerably. Whilst the study was unable to support health checks for participants, the men's narrative of declining physical fitness, constant fatigue and low immunity to infections were repeated amongst all but two of the participants. The paradox of these men's desires to restore their positions as family head and breadwinner lay in the fact that the decline in their physical health restricted them from returning to the types of physical work they had been performing previously. Re's admissions revealed this paradox in no uncertain terms:

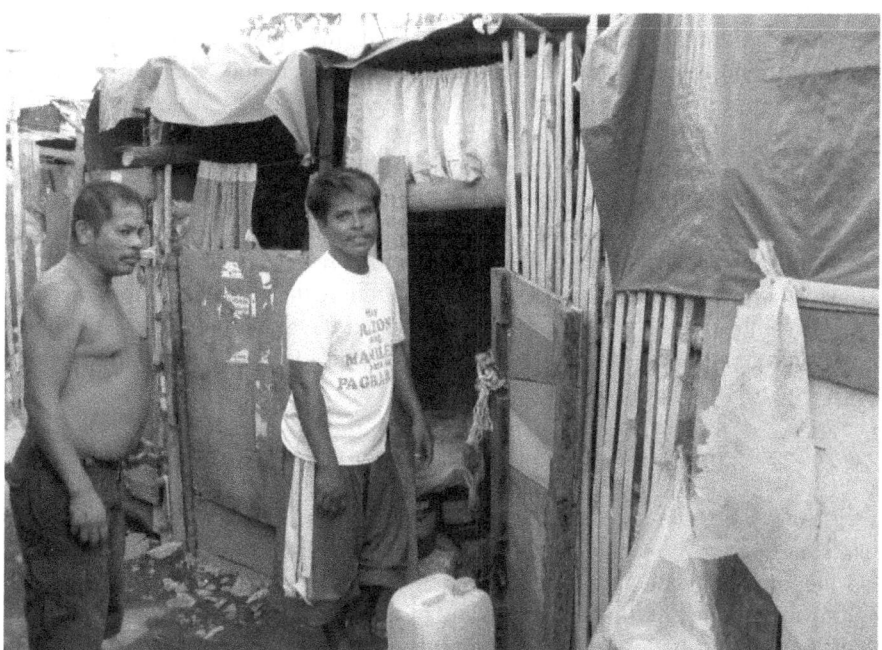

Figure 3.1   Al in front of his home in Baseco
Source: Author's own.

> I can't carry heavy loads anymore. The pain lasts for days if I take work as a
> cargador. It's impossible for me to continue this kind of work now. I've lost
> everything; my house, my business and my ability to work.

Courtenay (2000) has suggested that men in the United States often compromise
their health through performances of masculinity that rely on physical strength,
suffering and endurance of pain, making them less likely to engage in positive
health practices than women. This may also be true for some of the men in this
study who chose not to avail post-operative medical checks or drugs.[6]

---

6   Some of the men in the study were not given the option of post-operative care in
the short to medium term after discharge from the hospital. However other men were given
this option and all but one refused it. To what extent them men were acting out a particular
form of 'unhealthy behaviour … to demonstrate masculinity' (Courtenay, 2000, p. 1,390)
is unclear. Probing this subject with participants yielded an attitude of indifference that
I interpreted as primarily related to the self-perceived worthlessness of their own lives.
However the issue of follow-up health interventions for providers, both in Manila and other
sites, is worthy of more extensive analysis.

Whilst culturally embedded discourses of the male breadwinner figure prominently in Baseco men's constructions of masculinity through selling a kidney, in reflecting on my analysis of the men's narratives about the meaning and experience of this strategy, it alone seems an incomplete characterisation of the ways commercial kidney provision intersects with masculine ideals in the Philippines. Therefore I wish to now elaborate on the ways men manoeuvre and contest discourses of trafficking that situate them as 'victims', which I believe results in heightened self-constructions as contemporary 'heroes' of the Philippines. As far as I know, the question of how men manoeuvre these contradictions through culturally embedded bodily practices has escaped the attention of those studying organ trafficking and kidney sales in Manila, and indeed those studying human trafficking more generally.

Trafficking, Heroism and Bloodletting in Global Manila

If the male breadwinner model helps understand economically marginal Filipino men's motivations to sell a kidney, then how do they see themselves in the short and medium term after the transplantation? This question assumes a particular significance in the aftermath of the failure of the kidney sales of all the men in this study to secure a better future for themselves and their families and the related portrayal of their experiences through the media according to the victim discourse that is circulated within prevailing constructions of human trafficking. Manila's organ trade provides an exemplary site for the production of this victim rhetoric as trafficking as a way of defining these men's experiences has prevailed in both academic and popular writings about their experiences.

In their post-operative reflections on representations and relationships I found that Baseco's male kidney sellers began to engage in performances of heroism drawing on their experiences of selling a kidney as a central trope. Heroism as a theme in understanding recent expressions of Filipino masculinity has been discussed by McKay (2011) in his treatise on Filipino seafarers. In his analysis, 'Filipino seafarers have ... generally embraced the "hero" label ... combining providership with other traditionally masculine elements of heroism beyond the ability to (passively) suffer, such as: being physically tough, willing to take risks, and being adventurous and worthy' (2011, p. 7). The interpretation of heroism embraced by Baseco's kidney sellers is at once similar and different from that described by McKay in relation to seafarers. This is because the worldliness and adventurousness that comes with 'life on the high seas' as well as the official State discourse of heroism ascribed to all OFWs (overseas Filipino workers) (Guevarra, 2010), including seafarers are both absent for Baseco's kidney sellers. On the other hand, physical endurance and risk taking provide common ground for the construction of heroic masculinity amongst these two groups.

Nonetheless, although narratives of physical endurance and risk taking emerged within men's post-operative self-understandings, these are not the principal tenets of heroic masculinity upon which Baseco's male kidney providers drew. As

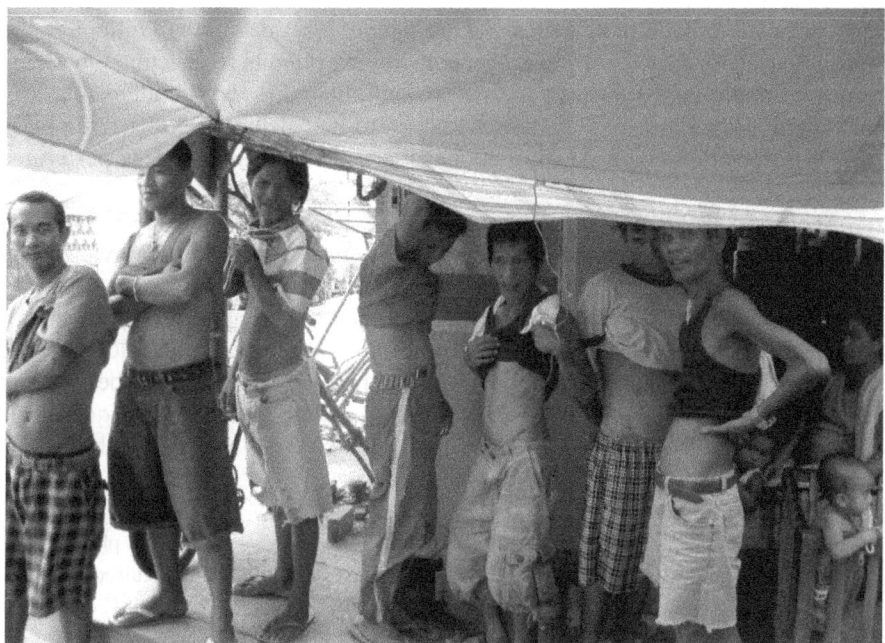

Figure 3.2   Participants parodying the 'spectacle' of the scar
Source: Author's own.

suggested above, performances of heroism for kidney providers are principally a response to the ways they are represented within popular discourses (primarily the media) and in particular the use of visual images that emphasise their scarred bodies (Figure 3.2). Responding to these post-operative representational outcomes the men in this study performed heroic masculinity principally through making visible their wounds/scars as significant embodied signs of sacrifice achieved through the culturally sanctioned medium of bloodletting. Unlike the expression of masculine ideals through other tenets of heroic masculinity, such as risk taking, bloodletting relates principally to religious and nationalist sacrifices for the nation. As Pingol (personal communication June 2010) reminds us, 'bloodletting is the first standard of Filipino masculinity'. Bloodletting has historically been associated with Filipino 'nationalist' heroes opposing foreign occupation (Spain, United States, Japan) of the Philippines and is inextricably linked to Filipino heroism interpreted as suffering and sacrificing for the nation (Rafael, 2000).[7] The

7   A study of role models amongst young people in the Philippines found that a large proportion of young men (28 per cent) identified Jose Rizal as their principle role model. The majority of young women identified their mothers (Sandoval et al., 1998). Jose Rizal (1861–1896) was a patriot and reformer during Spanish rule in the Philippines, writing

annual Easter crucifixion parades that are widely practiced in the Philippines are also intensely symbolic religious events involving pundits re-enactment of being crucified and paraded through the streets and involving very public displays of bloodletting. In short, bloodletting continues to be celebrated in the Philippines for its associations with deeply nationalistic and religious practices performed exclusively by men.

Whilst kidney providers in Baseco comply with media representations that represent them as victims of trafficking, by participating in interviews and photographs, such as the picture above, through discussions with them it became clear that they perceived these forums to be outlets through which to attempt to *celebrate* their status, thus subverting the victim narrative. The visible effects of the transplantations in the form of scars and healing wounds, they believe, act as significant bodily symbols of their sacrifice and as a scathing critique of the neoliberal impulse of global Manila that both creates their vulnerability and enables their exploitation. As Ge recounts:

> Many journalists have come to Baseco and interviewed us and taken our photos. Always the pose is the same; we must stand with our polos [shirts] raised and our scars visible. I don't mind doing this because other Filipinos will see the sacrifice that we have made. It's a physical sacrifice that should shame the government and so we must show our scars.

Despite their desire to engage in both critique of the Philippines contemporary development malaise, and the positive self-representations around their wounded bodies they hope to craft through their involvement in the media, the men ultimately do not have control over the production of narratives about their experiences that accompany these media exposes. These narratives emphasise the tragic victim rather than the sacrificial and suffering hero, thus leading men to negotiate another compromise to their efforts to recover a masculine sense of self.

Observations of their bodily conduct outside the sphere of the media during the field visits to Baseco revealed these alternative negotiations. In particular male kidney providers often walked around their neighbourhood with no upper garment or with their polo raised in the way it appears most commonly in the media. This, I believe, enables these men to participate more fully in the production of their own representations of their kidney sales. Further, for this study, the men suggested the 'staging' of their own version of the photo that typically appears in media stories. Some of the participants parodied the image by producing their own version in which they stood smiling as they raised their polos (see Figure 3.2).

It is important to attend to the production of discourses around trafficking that extend beyond those proffered by the media and in some academic accounts. This is necessary because it is revealing of the disjuncture that often exists between the

---

various treatise on reform and independence for the Philippines. He was executed in 1896, with the day of his execution celebrated annually as a national holiday in the Philippines.

narratives and meaning making processes of trafficked persons themselves and those put forward by external actors. In the case of Baseco's commercial kidney providers, the negotiations around representations of their experiences lead to new forms of bodily and spatial manoeuvring grounded in an everyday critique of the Philippines current development situation and the way bloodletting as heroic masculine practice figures in such a critique.

Discussion and Conclusions

In this chapter I have explored the gendered meanings attached to commercial kidney provision amongst men who are providers in Manila, the Philippines. This is in line with some recent scholarship on commercial transplantation that suggests that the meanings of these transactions for providers, though deeply embedded in economic imperatives associated with poverty and family insecurity, also extend beyond these concerns, at least for men. In my participants experiences economic marginality intersected with men's culturally sanctioned familial roles and with heroic ideals of masculinity within the Philippines, to produce a more fluid and, hopefully, temporally sensitive reading of both their motives in kidney selling and men's self-understandings post-transplantation.

Specifically, the narratives of these men revealed that while economic considerations figured prominently in their decisions to sell a kidney and post-transplantation trajectories, these considerations should to themselves be culturally embedded within discussions of longstanding masculine ideals in the Philippines. Traditional Filipino locus's of masculinity through heroism and the male breadwinner deserve more extensive treatment in understanding these men's decisions and experiences. In scholarly and popular accounts of human trafficking – both in the organ trade and other sectors where trafficking occurs – poverty is an oft-cited factor in explaining vulnerabilities that lead to trafficking, but rarely do accounts delve more deeply into this 'poverty-as-force' dialectic. How economic marginality relates to specific cultural contexts in informing decisions about livelihood options has, for example, been subject to very limited analysis for organ trafficking, and indeed human trafficking more generally. In this vein I wish to propose some further areas for consideration by those interested in the cultural and gendered logics of (male) bodies across borders.

For the men in this study, commercial organ provision represents a livelihood strategy and a means to restore and reconfigure their masculinity. In an important sense then, the sale of a kidney fulfils an economic and a symbolic function and must be understood within the broader context of Philippines current development malaise as it intersects with classed and gendered imaginaries. Simple accounts of exploitation of 'victims' whilst emotively powerful as devices to generate sympathy for the problem of trafficking, fail to capture these gendered meanings. Further, despite these men's desire to revive their masculinity through a kidney sale, commercial organ provision has contradictory outcomes for many Filipino men. First, money gains are often short term and health considerations diminish their working lives in the longer term. Second, their construction within popular discourses as victims of trafficking rails against their self-proclaimed masculine aspirations through kidney selling. These outcomes produce an engagement with Filipino notions of heroism as a means of at least partly reasserting these projects around masculinity.

In following the post-transplantation trajectories of men in this study, the failure of transplantation to fulfil their family livelihood and male breadwinner outcomes lead to attempts to recover some meaning from the experience. It is at this point that the discourse of the sacrificial hero came into play for the men in this study. Therefore we must be careful not to collapse various gendered and moral meanings of kidney provision for providers. For the men in this study new meanings were negotiated over time as their multiple losses (a kidney, the money, their health, and their assets) crystallised. In responding to these failed aspirations and concomitant media portrayals of the men as 'tragic victims', men's attribution of a moral meaning to their kidney sale oscillated away from the breadwinner model and towards heroic inscriptions. Masculinity is after all a social construct and is continually negotiated and performed in ways mediated by class, ethnicity, race, sexuality and circumstances (Hopkins, 2006).

Through my analysis I found current discussions of masculinity by geographers and in related disciplines wanting in one key respect. The literature suggests that the expression of masculinities amongst marginally-situated men occurs when these men draw on alternative (meaning non-hegemonic) constructions of masculinity, including those associated with violence, crime and (self-) harm. But these observations have generally been made in relation to men in Western contexts, rather than in the third world. Despite their socio-economic positions as slum dwellers in Manila, the men in this study drew on normative constructions of what it means to be a 'successful Filipino man' in creating social and gendered meanings from their experience of organ selling. At the same time, precisely because the element of exploitation is writ large in these experiences further manoeuvring also drawing on hegemonic ideals becomes necessary for these men. Following this it might be suggested that the explanatory potential of Connell's construct of 'hegemonic masculinity' is both useful and limited in this context. As has also been noted in Steve McKay's (2010, p. 2,011) discussion of Filipino men specifically and for Southeast Asian men more generally (Ford and Lyons, 2010) geographically extenuative research could deepen analyses of the complexities in (non)hegemonic masculinities in the third world. Yet the elaboration of these differences remains a largely unfulfilled task for geographers concerned with the interstices between masculinity, marginality and globalisation.

Further, consideration of a range of sites for the production of subaltern masculinity beyond the broad theme of migration/transnationality may also hold significant analytical potential in advancing discussions of masculinity in geography. The discussion in this chapter, specifically, has revealed commercial organ provision as both a livelihood strategy and a means of restoring a sense of a gendered selfhood, but with ambiguous consequences for Filipino men nonetheless.

Because men participate in Manila's kidney trade from a disadvantaged position and because the trade continues to operate in a clandestine manner, they are unable to negotiate appropriate short and long term medical care and, for most men, even basic post-operative check-ups. As a result men's health and subsequently their ability to work are diminished. The disjuncture between aspirations and outcomes for these men, paradoxically, can result in a further dilution of their sense of masculinity, rather than its restoration or even exacerbation within the contemporary milieu. Men's positions (and their negotiation of these) require a consideration of sites and themes beyond those that attend to migration and transnationality. Indeed, despite the Philippines being the largest and longest serving source of migrant labourers in Asia, including of men, a far greater proportion of marginal Filipino men negotiate the structures and relations of neoliberal globalisation from *within* the Philippines itself.

A final point for consideration here relates to the images, rather than actual parts, of bodies that move across borders. Discussion of the intersection between masculine notions of herosim and commercial organ provision in Manila demonstrate the spectacle inherent in the circulation of media images of scarred bodies and tragic narratives of 'trafficking victims' as they also move across borders (see also Yea, 2015, for a comparative discussion concerning the child trafficking victim). In this sense discussions in geography and elsewhere of bodies across borders could do well to engage with the ways discourses of the tragic victim can both dilute and lead to new negotiations of gendered meanings associated a range of forms of trafficking. Such undertakings could illuminate the multiple meanings associated with the sale of body parts that extend beyond the spectacle of the victim.

References

Aguilar, F. and Siruno, L., 2004. A Community Without a Kidney: A tragedy? Analysis of the moral and ethical aspects of organ kidney donation. In: D.R.J. Macer, ed. 2004. *Challenges for Bioethics in Asia*. [online] Available at: <http://www.eubios.info/abc5bk.htm> [Accessed 22 May 2014].

Andrijasevic, R., 2007. The Spectacle of Misery. Gender, migration and representation in anti-trafficking campaigns. *Feminist Review*, 86, pp. 24–44.

Asia ACTS, no date. The Philippines: Fifth organ trafficking hotspot. [online] Available at: <http://www.humantraffickinginasia.net/databank/20080331> [Accessed 1 November 2011].

Bagayaua, G., 2009. Organ Trade Continues Despite Ban on Transplants to Foreigners. *ABS-CBN News*. 8 March. [online] Available at: <http://www.abs-cbnnews.com/special-report/03/08/09/organ-trade-continues-despite-ban-transplantation-foreigners> [accessed 22 March 2010].

Beeks, K., and Amir, D., eds., 2006. *Trafficking and the Global Sex Industry*. Lanham: Lexington Books.

Brennan, D., 2005. Methodological Challenges in Research with Trafficked Persons: Tales from the field. *International Migration*, 43(1/2), pp. 35–54.

Carney, S., 2011. *The Red Market: On the trail of the world's organ brokers, bone thieves, blood farmers and child traffickers*. New York: William Marrow.

Connell, R.W., 1992. Masculinity, Violence and War. In: M.S. Kimmel and M.A. Messner, eds. 1992. *Men's lives*. Second edition. New York: Macmillan, pp. 176–83.

———, 1995. *Masculinities*. Berkeley: University of California Press.

Courtenay, W.H, 1999. Youth Violence? Let's call it what it is. *Journal of American College Health*, 48(3), pp. 141–2.

———, 2000. Constructions of Masculinity and their Influence on Men's Well-Being: A theory of gender and health. *Social Science and Medicine*, 50, pp. 1,385–401.

Courtenay, W. and Sabo, D., 2001. Preventative Health Strategies for Men in Prison. In: D. Sabo, T. Kupers and W. London, eds. 2001. *Confronting Prison Masculinities: The gendered politics of punishment*. Philadelphia: Temple University Press, pp. 157–72.

Crowley-Matoka, M. and Lock, M., 2006. Organ Transplantation in a Globalised World. *Mortality*, 11(2), pp. 166–81.

Datta, K., McIlwaine, C., Herbert, J., Evans, Y., May, J. and Wills, J. 2009. Men On the Move: Narratives of migration and work among low-paid migrant men in London. *Social and Cultural Geography*, 10(8), pp. 853–73.

Dimetriou, D., 2001. Connell's Concept of Hegemonic Masculinity: A critique. *Theory and Society*, 30(3), pp. 337–61.

Doezema, J., 2010. *Sex Slaves and Discourse Masters: The construction of trafficking*. London and New York: Routledge.

Ehrenreigh, B. and Hochschild, A.R. eds., 2004. *Global Woman: Nannies, maids and sex workers in the new economy*. New York: Henry Holt.

Ford, M. and Lyons, L., 2011. Introduction. In: M. Ford and L. Lyons, eds. 2001. *Men and Masculinities in Southeast Asia*. London: Routledge, pp. 1–29.

Gagaloc, R., 2008. NBI Raises Alarm on Child-Organ Trafficking. ABS-CBN News, 24 August. [online] Available at: <http://unionssaynotochildlabor.com/nbi-raises-alarm-on-child-organ-trafficking/> [Accessed 12 March 2010].

Guevarra, A., 2010. *Marketing Dreams, Manufacturing Heroes: The transnational labour brokering of Filipino workers*. New Brunswick, NJ: Rutgers University Press.

Hamdy, S., 2010. The Organ Transplant Debate in Egypt: A social anthropological analysis. *Droit et cultures*, 59, pp. 357–65.

Herbert, J., 2008. Masculinity and Migration: Life stories of East African men. In: L. Ryan and W. Webster, eds. 2008. *Gendering Migration: Masculinity, femininity and ethnicity in post-war Britain*. Aldershot: Ashgate Publishing, pp. 189–204.

Hochschild, A., 2009. Childbirth at the Global Crossroads. *The American Prospect*. [online] Available at: <http://www.prospect.org/cs/articles?article=childbirth_at_the_global_crossroads> [Accessed 21 March 2010].

Hopkins, P., 2006. Youthful Muslim Masculinities: Gender and generational relations. *Transactions of the Institute of British Geographers*, 31, pp. 337–52.

———, 2007. Young People, Masculinities, Religion and Race: New social geographies. *Progress in Human Geography*, 31, pp. 163–77.

Hua, J. and Nigorizawa, N., 2010. US Sex Trafficking, Women's Human Rights and the Politics of Representation. *International Feminist Journal of Politics*, 12 (3/4), pp. 401–23.

Hung, C.T., 2005. Globalization as a Gender Strategy: Respectability, masculinity, and convertibility across the Vietnamese diaspora. In: R.P. Appelbaum and I. Robinson, eds. 2005. *Critical globalization studies*. London: Routledge, pp. 313–32.

Jackson, P., Stevenson, N. and Brooks, K., 1999. Black Male: Advertising and the cultural politics of masculinity. *Gender, Place and Culture*, 1, pp. 49–59.

Kierans, C., 2011. Anthropology, Organ Transplantation and the Immune System: Resituating commodity and gift exchange. *Social Science and Medicine*, 73, pp. 1,469–76.

Kupar, R., 2002. The Tragedy of the Victim Rhetoric: Resurrecting the 'native' subject in international/post-colonial legal politics. *Harvard Human Rights Journal*, 15(Spring), pp. 1–37.

Lainez, N., 2010. Representing Sex Trafficking in Southeast Asia? The victim staged. In: T. Zheng, ed. 2010. *Sex Trafficking, Human Rights and Social Justice*. New York: Routledge, pp. 134–49.

Longhurst, R., 2000. Geography and Gender: Masculinities, Male Identity and Men. *Progress in Human Geography*, 24(3), pp. 439–44.

May, J., Datta, K., Evans, Y., Herbert, J. and McIlwaine, C., 2008. Travelling Neoliberalism: Polish and Ghanaian migrant workers in London. In: A. Smith, A. Stenning and K. Willis, eds. 2008. *Social justice and neoliberalism: Global perspectives*. New York: Verso, pp. 61–81.

McDowell, L., 2003. *Redundant Masculinities? Employment change and white working class youth*. Oxford: Blackwell.

McKay, S., 2010. 'So They Remember Me When I'm Gone': Remittances, fatherhood and gender relations in the Philippines. Unpublished paper.

———, 2011. Re-Masculinising the Hero: Filipino migrant men and gender privilege. Asia Research Institute (ARI) Working Paper, No. 172. ARI, National University of Singapore, Singapore (December).

Mendoza, R.L., 2010. Price Deflation and the Underground Organ Economy in the Philippines. *Journal of Public Health*, 2010, pp. 1–7.

Messerschmidt, J.W., 1993. *Masculinities and Crime: Critique and reconceptualisation of theory*. Lanham, MD: Rowman and Littlefield.

Messner, M.A. and Sabo, D., 1994. *Sex, Violence and Power in Sports: Rethinking masculinity*. Freedom, CA: The Crossing Press.

Oakley, A., 1981. Interviewing Women: A contradiction in terms. In: H. Roberts, ed. 1981. *Doing Feminist Research.* London: Routledge and Kegan Paul, pp. 30–61.

Osella, F. and Osella, C., 1999. Migration, Money and Masculinity in Kerala. *Journal of the Royal Anthropological Institute,* 6, pp. 117–33.

Pajnik, M., 2010. Media Framing of Trafficking. *International Feminist Journal of Politics,* 12(1), pp. 45–64.

Parrenas, R., 2008. Transnational Fathering: Gendered conflicts, distant disciplining and emotional gaps. *Journal of Ethnic and Migration Studies,* 37(4), pp. 1,057–72.

Parry, B., 2008. Entangled Exchange: Reconceptualising the characterisation and practice of bodily commodification. *Geoforum,* 39, pp. 1,133–44.

Pingol, A.T., 2001. *Remaking Masculinities: Identity, power and gender dynamics in families with migrant wives and househusbands.* Quezon City: University Centre for Women's Studies, University of the Philippines.

Pribilsky, J., 2012. Consumption Dilemmas: Tracking masculinity, money and transnational fatherhood between Ecuadorian Andes and New York City. *Journal of Ethnic and Migration Studies,* 38(2), pp. 323–43.

Rafael, V., 2000. *White Love and Other Events in Filipino History.* Durham and London: Duke University Press Republic of the Philippines, 2003. Anti-Trafficking in Persons Act, Republic Act 9208, Congress of the Philippines, Metro Manila. [online] Available at: <http://www.lawphil.net/statutes/repacts/ra2003/ra_9208_2003.html> [Accessed 27 May 2010].

Rubio, R. and Green, R.J., 2009. Filipino Masculinity and Psychological Distress: A preliminary comparison between gay and heterosexual men. *Sexuality Research and Social Policy,* 6(3), pp. 61–75.

Sanal, A., 2011. *New Organs Within Us: Transplantation and the moral economy.* North Carolina: Duke University Press.

Sandoval, G., Mangahas, M. and Guevarra, L.L., 1998. Gender and Young People's Role Models in the Philippines. In: ISA (International Sociological Association). *14th World Congress of Sociology.* Montreal, Canada, August.

Scheper-Hughes, N., 2000. The Global Traffic in Human Organs. *Current Anthropology,* 41(2), pp. 191–211.

———, 2003. Rotten Trade: Millennial capitalism, human values, and global justice in organs trafficking. *Journal of Human Rights,* 2(2), pp. 197–226.

———, 2004. Parts Unknown: Undercover ethnography of the organs-trafficking underworld. *Ethnography,* 5, pp. 29–71.

———, 2008. Illegal Organ Trade: Global justice and the traffic in organs. In: R. Gruessner and E. Benedetti, eds. 2008. *Living organ donor transplantation.* New York: McGraw-Hill, pp. 106–21.

———, 2011. Mr Tati's Holiday and Joao's Safari: Seeing the world through transplant tourism. *Body and Society,* 17 (2/3), pp. 55–92.

Scheyvens, R. and Leslie, H., 2000. Gender, Ethics and Empowerment: Dilemmas of development fieldwork. *Women's Studies International Forum*, 23(1), pp. 119–30.

Shimazono, Y., 2008. Repaying and Cherishing the Gift of Life: Gift exchange and living related kidney transplantation in the Philippines. *Anthropology in Action*, 15(3), pp. 34–46.

Surtees, R., 2008. Trafficked men as unwilling victims. *St Anthony's International Review*, 4(1), pp. 16–36.

———, 2011. *Trafficked to Sea. The exploitation of Ukrainian seafarers and fishermen.* Geneva: IOM and NEXUS Institute.

Townsend, N., 2002. *The Package Deal: Marriage, Work and Fatherhood in Men's Lives.* Philadelphia: Temple University Press.

United Nations, 2000. *Protocol to Prevent, Suppress and Punish Trafficking in Persons, Especially Women and Children.* Vienna: UNODC (United Nations Office on drugs and Crime).

World Health Organisation (WHO), 2003. *WHO Ethical and Safety Recommendations for Interviewing Trafficked Women.* Geneva: WHO.

Yea, S., 2010. Trafficking in part(s): the commercial kidney market in a manila slum. *Global Social Policy*, 10(3), pp. 358–76.

———, 2015. 'Girls on Film: Affective Politics and the Creation of an Intimate Anti-Trafficking Public in Singapore through Film Screenings', *Political Geography*, 45: 45–54.

———, 2014. 'Troubled Waters: The Trafficking of Filipino Fishermen on Long Haul Fishing Boats through Singapore'. Report for TWC2, Singapore.

Chapter 4

A Bull Market? Devices of Qualification and Singularisation in the International Marketing of US Sperm

Bronwyn Parry

Introduction

In April 2012, *Time* magazine undertook an analysis of the dramatic acceleration of international demand for human sperm that had been banked in the United States, noting, in an article entitled 'Frozen Assets' that the export of this commodity has recently become 'what financial analysts call a growth sector in the American economy – one of the few in which the U.S. is running a significant trade surplus' (Newton-Small, 2012, p. 34). As Rene Almeling (2011) noted in her recent analysis of the commodification of gametes, the historical preference for use of 'fresh semen' in assisted reproduction did not decline until the 1980s when the AIDS epidemic gave a fillip to the practice of banking sperm by reducing transmission risks through quarantining. Since then, commercial banking of sperm has grown into an extremely lucrative business. Citing information gleaned from MarketData industry analysis, *Time* reports that the largest sperm bank in the world (and in the US) California Cryobank recorded sales of 23 million US dollars in 2011 within a sector with total sales in excess of 100 million US dollars. Export occupies an important niche in the marketing strategy of such banks. The world's (and the US's) largest sperm bank, California Cryobank, and New York's Fairfax Cryobank both report that over 10 per cent of their sales are exports. The next largest US bank, Xytex Cryo, has the strongest international presence conducting more than 30 per cent of its business abroad. In 2005 ABC news reported that the top four US sperm banks together controlled 65 per cent of the global market, exporting to over sixty countries worldwide.

Why should sperm from the US prove to be so desirable to international consumers? It might be presumed that this is simply an artefact of the phenomenon of economies of scale. US banks are bigger, have larger quantities of more ethnically diverse stock, which, combined with sophisticated technologies for storing and transporting these gametes generates an unrivalled capacity to circulate their product within the global reproductive marketplace in the most cost effective manner. This argument has some substance. However, it is also true that many other well respected banks exist in European countries; in Canada, Australia, the

Far East and in South Africa and South America (all countries to which American sperm is now exported) that are perfectly capable of supplying domestic demand for donated sperm without resort to importation. Why then has American sperm become such a desirable commodity? What sets of interests and concerns animate this trade and why is it important to understand them?

In order to address these questions I begin by analysing how the global circulation of reproductive materials first became possible, paying particular attention to the historiography of the development of its usage as a bankable commodity. This has its genesis not only in the history of medicine, as might be imagined, but also in the history of selective breeding in agriculture where its application was informed by two fixations that, I believe, continue to animate contemporary engagements with assisted human reproduction: husbandry and pedigree. As I shall demonstrate shortly, the question of why US sperm banks have come to so dominate these international markets can be answered, in part, by reference to variances in the regulation of tissue banking in different national jurisdictions. But this is not the whole story. For here I want to argue that a different metric is at work, one that has enabled American sperm to become 'qualified' to use the Michel Callon's term, that is to say, singularised in relation to its competitors, in such a way that it is favourably evaluated and judged as preferable.

The metric through which this qualification is achieved is one of *characterisation* delivered, as I shall argue, through the mechanism of advanced donor profiling. The genealogical connection between profiling and its historical counterpart, pedigree, will be excavated in order to show how profiling ushers in a new iteration of a *régime ancien* in which a range of attributes are valorised and employed to rank individuals and to position them eugenically within cohorts that, as Barney (2005, p. 212) suggests, 'represent the social elite rather than the general population'. The chapter examines the emergent forms of 'bio-sociality' to which these metrics give rise (Rabinow, 1992) by investigating how, and in what ways, they are informed by what Hacking calls the 'genetic imperative' (Hacking, 2006, p. 89) – the need to categorise our lives according to genetic inferences about human traits. It concludes by considering how the technological ability to engineer these traits through assisted conception is now driving the development of a global market for 'prime' reproductive resources, and, in so doing, sedimenting a biologised vision of society and set of attendant practices that serves only to privilege the reproduction of these imaginary 'biosocial elites'.

Frogs in Britches: The Emergence of *Artificial Fecundation*

Artificial insemination (AI) – the introduction of semen into the vagina or cervix of a female by any means other than sexual intercourse – is not, in any sense, a new practice. The impression that it is derives, in part, from the presumption that the practise has been employed in qualitatively different ways, or for distinctive purposes, in particular realms: in animal husbandry and human conception, for example. Many contemporary accounts of assisted conception thus begin in the early twentieth century with vignettes that focus on the first attempts to achieve pregnancy in women through impregnation with donor sperm. By not contextualising these developments within the longer durée of experiments in assisted reproduction in animals (which underpinned the later expansion and commercialisation of advanced human invitro fertilisation and insemination techniques) an opportunity is lost to trace how the particular philosophies, postulations and values that informed those earlier practices continue to shape the organisation and administration of the commercial assisted conception industry, to this day. To understand how it become possible to intervene in reproduction and how this capacity was then deployed in the political enterprise of selective breeding we must return, at first, to the middle of the seventeenth century.

It was here, in Amsterdam, in 1672 that the celebrated Dutch naturalist Jan Swammerdam began experiments to investigate one of the most vexatious and unresolved questions of the day – how animals were generated. In what was then an astounding demonstration, he dissected a silkworm peeling back the outer skin to reveal beneath the tightly coiled wings and limbs of a moth lying in a state of suspended animation, awaiting only its appointed hour to unfold into life. The experiment was thought to provide evidence in support of the theory of preformation – the idea that every living creature contains already within it another of the same species – as one finds, for example, a miniature navel orange growing already within another. This unfolding, it was thought, would occur spontaneously sparked by what other like-minded adherents of preformation, such as Buffon and Needham, described as a generative or 'vegetative force', something akin to the Aristotelian notion of an '*aura seminalis*'.

Unconvinced by these assertions the Italian priest Lazzaro Spallanzani began an alternative line of enquiry, furthering earlier studies on the role of seminal fluid in conception through experimentation with frogs. Building on Leeuwenhoek's prior discovery that the fluid contained 'spermatic worms', Spallanzani determined to 'follow this race of little animals to the end' (Pinto-Correia, 1997, p. 62). In order to establish whether frogs eggs could develop by themselves he conducted many experiments to collect seminal fluid including famously clothing many dozens of excited male frogs in tight waxed taffeta britches. Having secured the 'liquor' through such ingenious methods he then performed a number of trials proving its essential role in conception by demonstrating that only eggs that had been bought into direct contact with it 'bought forth young' (Pinto-Correia, 1997, p. 199). More significant perhaps than even this was his realisation that he could intervene in this process serving as the instrument through which the intermingling could be effected. Taking the isolated semen from within the britches and placing it near to the frogs eggs did not result in conception, however, his touching it upon the eggs invariably did. What he was to later describe as the practice of 'artificial fecundation' which succeeded, as he noted 'as well as if the male had performed his proper function' (Pinto- Correia, 1997, p. 197) was further refined in his later experiments. Having injected a spaniel bitch with sperm derived from another dog of the same breed, he was astonished to note that his intervention culminated, 62 days later, in the production of three lively pups.

As Clara Pinto-Correia notes in her fascinating account of this work it is important to draw careful distinctions between the kinds of techniques Spallanzani was employing in such experiments. Although he described all these interventions as 'impregnations' his intermediations with frogs (where fertilisation is external) would now be described as constituting a form of invitro fertilisation. In the case of the spaniel, fertilisation was internal as the sperm was introduced into the female's body. It thus constitutes the first documented instance of what we now term 'artificial insemination'. Both techniques were however, united by their demonstration of the fact that sperm could be deployed out with the body or, more specifically, that its vitality and fecundity could be sustained (in certain controlled environmental conditions) such that it could be mobilised for use over space and time.

Spallanzani attempted to further prolong the viability of the collected sperm by enclosing semen in glass vessels immersed in freezing mixtures of rock salt and ice (recorded at minus 17 degrees on the Réaumur scale or minus 21 degrees Celsius) and spirits of nitre at temperatures of minus 24°Ré or minus 30°C. Surprisingly, some of the sperm survived the freezing process, and moreover, retained its regenerative properties, albeit, not for long. In 1866 Mantegazza, an Italian naturalist, repeated Spallanzanni's experiments reporting survival at temperatures of minus 17 degrees Celsius. However it was not until Faraday, Cailletet and Pictet's successful liquefaction of what were then considered to be permanent gases such as oxygen and nitrogen that research into cryogenics, including the preservation of tissues at ultra-low temperatures,[1] was formalised. As I have noted elsewhere, (Parry, 2004) despite these advances the most significant breakthroughs in cryobiology did not occur until the early 1930s, some by serendipitous accident. Inspired by experiments undertaken at Leiden from 1908–1935 by the French biologist Paul Becquerel, Basil Luyet, another Jesuit priest and naturalist, began to undertake systematic studies of the effects of ultra-low temperatures on the survival rates of frog spermatozoa. In seeking to explain how the thawed sperm could retain its motility and vitality Luyet speculated that it could be due to the metabolic substrate of sperm (fructose) acting as a protective media.

This research sparked considerable interest in the role that cryoprotectants could play in reducing or eliminating the damaging effects of freezing injuries on tissues, notably at the National Institute for Medical Research Laboratory at Mill Hill in London. It was here that post-thaw sperm motility rates in excess of 50 per cent were first achieved, albeit through unanticipated means: the accidental substitution of a fixative, glycerol, with the usual cryopreservative, bought about when a lab technician wrongly reapplied labels that had fallen off bottles of each. Despite the unconventional methodology the identification and use of glycerol as a cryoprotectant revolutionised the practice of storing mammalian cells enabling them

---

1   Oxygen liquefies at minus 183°C for example.

to be archived for years without loss of vitality. This, in turn, fundamentally altered the historical dynamics of the cellular life cycle by enabling tissues, but in particular gametes, to become detached and disassociated from the bodies that produced them. Immortalisation liberated them, freeing them to take up their own trajectory, their own 'career' as Appadurai would call it, one that begins with their deposition within a kind of artificial body: an environmentally controlled, long-term and secure repository for this newly exploitable reproductive material – the gamete bank.

Bull Markets: The Globalisation of Trade in Sperm

It might be assumed that it is a simple pathway from here to the development of the contemporary human sperm banks that are the subject of this chapter. However, trajectories are rarely perfectly parabolic or indeed singular. The story of the development and use of banked sperm in artificial insemination takes here an interesting deviation, one that provides some important insights into the way such practices have evolved over time: the technologies and economic imperatives that have facilitated their routinisation and later globalisation, and the preoccupations that have shaped the ways in which they been adopted, and are regulated, in particular settings. For, as we shall see, artificial insemination operates in a number of registers simultaneously and some interesting points of intersection can be discerned between them. The story of its usage as a bankable commodity has its genesis, for example, not in the human population but rather in the history of selective breeding practices in domestic, but primarily agricultural animals. Its usage in this domain has been animated by two concepts that prove to have strong resonances in contemporary practices of human artificial insemination and sperm banking: husbandry and pedigree.

It was here, in the world of livestock production and improvement, that the potential of AI was first recognised and models for cost efficient adoption first generated. Translating AI from the laboratory bench to commercial production was achieved through the introduction of new techniques but also novel uses of existing transportation networks. Contrary to popular belief, these experiments were not, initially, very high tech. The first international transportation of sperm occurred in 1925 when rabbit semen was posted from Cambridge to Edinburgh, amazingly, surviving the night train to effect fertilisation the following day (Bowman, p. 16). The economic and geographic scaling up of the enterprise which followed, was dependent not on the development of more sophisticated techniques of insemination, for these remained fairly consistent over time, but rather on the development of air travel and other globalising forces – including corporate consolidation.

Reviewing the historiography of the cattle breeding industry, in which AI now plays a central role, provides some important insights into the factors that motivated the early adoption of this technique and how these were promoted by its advocates. Key amongst these was its perceived capacity to facilitate, accelerate and expedite the practice of animal husbandry, of breeding for selected characteristics. Its proponents were very quick to recognise, as Bowman puts it, the extraordinary potential of 'what might be termed the whole package of "AI" and all that is made possible through the widespread use of the technique [including] marked economies of scale for the famers in the costs of cattle breeding, the identification of superior sires and their subsequent extended use, and the more effective control of certain cattle diseases' (Bowman, p. ii). These elements were, of course, interdependent. Superior sires included not only those identified through the use of extensive genealogical pedigrees as most 'valuable' but which were also, necessarily, free of disease; intensive use of which could, at least in theory, maximise intergenerational productivity and reliability of the herd and its maintenance. Commitment to the principle of selective breeding for enhanced performance was thus a prime objective of those involved in promotion of this technique. So, for example, the first AI equipment to be introduced to the UK was imported by Sir John Hammond and Danish veterinarian Eduard Sorensen both of whom were centrally involved in the Samso Elite Cattle Breeding Programme (Bowman, p. 11).[2]

The realisation that AI could enable 'superior' bulls to be used 'extensively' – in both a geographic and genetic sense – spurred efforts to find new methods of transporting semen from such animals internationally. There was a sudden recognition that 'the potential use of valuable males could be increased if semen could be kept successfully for longer periods and transported to females some distance away, and, be made available at the optimum time in the female's oestrus cycle' (Bowman, p. 16). Consequently in the spring of 1937 bull semen was sent to and from Holland and England for the first time via Royal Dutch Airlines. It remained, for the most part, suitable for insemination, despite the vicissitudes of distance and the insults of the freezing and thawing process leading the protagonists to conclude that cross border insemination was indeed 'a feasible proposition' (Edwards, p. 507).

Use of AI became routinised amongst dairy farmers in the Scandinavia and the UK in the 1950s, with demand driven by smallholders who paid just one pound for semen from a bull that would otherwise have cost them £1,500 to buy and maintain. By 1958, 90 percent of all dairy cows in Denmark were artificially inseminated (Bowman, p. 12). Uptake intensified equally dramatically in post war Britain.[3] The cryogenic storage of the semen also secured another very important achievement; one that I want to focus on for the rest of this chapter as I return to the realm of human sperm banking. It enabled sperm to be hierachised and marketed in qualitatively different ways to how it had been historically, providing consumers (in this case, farmers) with access to stock that superseded anything available locally, or even temporally. Bowman provides a detailed account of the

---

2   This was a Danish programme designed to produce an elite herd through highly selective breeding performed using AI.

3   Rising in Somerset, for example, from 1388 inseminations in 1944 to 31,592 in 1947 (Bowman, p. 59).

impact that cryogenics had on practice and marketing within animal husbandry and it is worth reproducing here as it foregrounds so well the kinds of ontological and practical shifts in orientation that have also since come to animate contemporary human sperm banking. As she explains:

> Perhaps the most significant technical development in the AI service since its inception has been the introduction of deep freeze storage of semen, for it is this that has enabled centres to offer a more comprehensive choice of bulls. In the early days semen could only be stored successfully for a matter of days. Consequently it was usually only possible for a farmer to obtain semen from a bull standing at the nearest AI centre. This obviously imposed fairly strict limits on choice. Now by means of long term storage, in addition to 'bull-of-the-day semen' from an increased variety of breeds … centres also offer a nomination service. On payment of an extra fee farmers may nominate and reserve semen from a specific bull. These include especially rated 'premium sires' with high estimated values. Nominated bulls may not be standing at the local centre and may not even still be alive … (Bowman, p.13).

Devices for Commodifying, Qualifying and Singularising Human Sperm

In outlining some of the reasons why individuals engage in forms of cross border reproductive care, Gürtin and Inhorn (2011) note that an important driver is the heterogeneity of legal frameworks that govern assisted reproductive technologies in different national jurisdictions, which are more or less permissive. These distinctions create an uneven regulatory landscape, one that would-be consumers, who are prevented from accessing care due to ethical or legal prohibitions in their own countries, are able to exploit. To date most attention has been focused on how differences in regulation affect the provision of care offered to particular constituencies (such as lesbian parents for example). However, regulatory inconsistencies also play a very significant, though as yet largely undocumented, role in shaping the ways in which reproductive 'products' are marketed in particular jurisdictions. In seeking to explain why US sperm has become such a desirable export commodity it is essential to understand why individuals select it, in preference to other like commodities to which they may also have access.

The sociologist Michel Callon and colleagues argue in the paper 'The Economy of Qualities' (Callon et al., 2002) that if we are to understand the structures of competition that exist within, and shape markets, we must pay attention to the role that dynamics of similitude and dissimilitude play. In seeking to make their product more desirable than any other, producers must first 'singularise' it in relation to its competitors. This 'singularisation of a product' is obtained they argue (p. 203) 'against a background of similitude – the difference that enables a product to capture the consumer always involves the prior assertion of a resemblance which suggests an association between the consumer's former attachments and the new ones proposed'. In other words in undertaking this process of singularisation much is to be gained by at first acknowledging the consumers' interest in, and attachment to, the general species of a product before providing them with a suitable means of discerning the superiority of the one proffered by a particular producer. But how can consumers manage to grasp differences when products are so similar? As they go on to suggest, this is achieved in part through the complex work that the producer undertakes to characterise and qualify products in ways that encourage consumers to evaluate them positively in relationship to available competitors. Many material and informational devices are called upon to perform this work: packaging, advertising and testing are all enjoined to help in the process of characterising the product as superior in the mind of the consumer.

This thesis can be usefully employed to shed light on the question of why and how the international market for sperm has become so differentiated and hierachised and how products are singularised within it. Regulation, it would seem, could be added here as another material device that is employed to qualify US sperm as a more desirable product than others in the global marketplace. It does so by positioning it in relationship to its competitors in ways that serve to construct it, from the consumer's point of view at least, as a superior product to that available locally. This is achieved in two ways. Firstly, unlike rival products (in this case sperm that is available to consumers in their domestic banks), the semen stored in many privatised US cryobanks can be fully anonymised. As Dennison (2007) and others have noted many countries, including Canada, the Netherlands, Australia, Sweden and Austria have now prohibited anonymised sperm donation in the interests of assuring the child's right to know their biological parentage. The UK's Human Fertilisation and Embryology Authority (HFEA) also determined in 2004 that the identity of donors who bank sperm in the UK must be disclosed to their offspring at the age of 18. These new regulations resulted in a well-documented downturn in donations and a complete prohibition of use of anonymised sperm in these localities. As Turkmendag et al. (2008, p. 284) note, this generated scarcity within domestic sperm markets created (in the minds of recipients, at least) a 'pressure to accept donors with suboptimal characteristics', to endure long waiting lists, or alternatively to embrace the use of imported cryogenically stored sperm.

Another important regulatory distinction relates to restrictions that are placed on the number of children that can be conceived from an individual donor. Under the UK's Human Fertilisation and Embryology Act (1990) no donor may create more than 10 families. No legislation of this kind exists in the US and sperm banks are, consequently, largely self-regulated. The Federal Drug Administration controls circulation of human tissue (and hence gametes) but does not require sperm banks to place limits on births to individual donors or even to report or track numbers of live births from donations. Some cryobanks have become signatories to codes of conduct developed by industry associations such as the American Society of Reproductive Medicine which propose a limit of 25 live births per sperm donor; however, adherence to such standards remains voluntary and is not monitored. One aspect of 'product development' that *is* very tightly regulated in the US gamete market is what might be termed 'quality control'. As Pi notes (2009, p. 379), the FDA's regulation of sperm banking in the US primarily focuses on 'donor screening, quality processing, and record keeping with the goal of keeping infectious tissue out of circulation'. Infectious tissue in this context includes sperm that might test positive for HIV and hepatitis. All sperm donations are thus quarantined for six months prior to being released for use.

What this analysis reveals is how the unevenness and inconsistent approach to regulation of sperm banking at state and federal levels within the US (which has allowed many to operate without robust oversight or accountability) has, ironically, served to generate a product that is presented to consumers as both biologically safer and more socially 'unencumbered' than that which may be available in their own jurisdictions. Whilst in advanced economies, such as the UK, testing regimes are commensurate with those instituted by the FDA, in other countries they are not, making US sperm a more desirable product. Anonymity provides another important point of singularisation: for some consumers not having to admit of the donor's identity frees them from any obligation to the maintenance of kinship relations over time, another 'unique selling point' for US sperm.

Advanced Donor Profiling: Pedigree and the Hierarchisation of Donors

Whilst regulation proves an important material device for 'singularising' US sperm within the international market place, its role is overshadowed by the work of another mechanism that I believe plays an even more pivotal role: advanced donor profiling. Qualification is here secured through a direct appeal to 'quality' itself; in fact, I would argue, by reference to what is actively constructed as 'pedigree'. Space precludes a more detailed examination of the many kinds of profiles that banks produce but a brief analysis that contrasts those available in the US with those typically available from public and privately funded banks in the UK (and in many other countries) may, at least, serve to demonstrate some of the dramatic incommensurabilities that exist in the way the pedigrees of particular donors are constructed and represented in these jurisdictions.

Taking the donor profiles offered by the London Sperm Bank (now the UK's largest sperm bank) by way of example, we see that their catalogues offer only very basic information about the donor. This is typologised in three ways; General Information: ethnic origin, race, nationality, religion, education and occupation; Physical Attributes: height, weight, eye colour, hair colour and skin tone and Personality: which outlines interests, hobbies and skills. The information provided in each category is very minimal, typically comprising only a single word or phrase such as: British, MSc Biology, Blonde, Music, Diving or Multilingual. This may also be supplemented by a few sentences that comprise the staff's 'impression of the donor' and a few words on their medical history: typically, blood type or presence of particular conditions such as asthma or eczema (although donors are also routinely tested medically and genetically for a range of conditions).

Consumers who have registered for treatment at associated fertility clinics are able to purchase vials online (add to cart) having made their selection on the basis of this information.

In stark contrast to this, donors on the US's most popular banking sites are characterised, which is also to say, in Callonistic terms, 'qualified', with what could only be described as an exceptionally fine degree of calibration. Basic donor profiles here provide all the information offered by UK banks including a family medical history, a 'personal essay' penned by the donor that describes his motivations and sense of self and a staff impression of the donor. If we imagine though, following Callon et al., that a product is not a static object but rather a process (a continually evolving sequence of transformations) then it perhaps most useful to think of it as primarily 'a negotiation' one that is continually revisited by all those actors involved in its design, production, distribution and consumption. The aim of this negotiation is to position it in 'a space of goods – in a system of differences and similarities, of distinct yet connected categories' (Callon et al., 2002, p. 198) – a space that makes comparisons possible. Although it may appear so this is not a case, however, of simply making information that already exists about the characteristics of particular products/donors visible – it is rather about firstly defining and then objectifying those characteristics that are to be 'valued'. This as Callon et al. (2002, p. 199) suggest, involves what they term 'specific metrological work and heavy investments in measuring equipment' notably, in the domains of testing and packaging.

When commercial sperm banking first began in the US in the 1970s profiles were, as they are now in the UK and other countries, rather scant, containing only very basic information about the donor. As the domestic and international marketplace for donor sperm has become more competitive, and hence, more crowded, US providers have begun, in conversation with their consumers and producers, to together construct much more sophisticated material devices for manufacturing, objectively testing and packaging the 'pedigree' of each donor. The 'extended donor profile' provides a detailed three generation medical history and a battery of genetic tests. Other instruments such as Keirsey test results are used to 'verify' the donor's personality traits, behavioural profile and temperament; whilst Facial Features reports and Donor Matching services are used to classify and correlate anatomical features. Childhood Photo packages, recorded Donor Conversations and Express Yourself reports (where offered by the donor) are also made available to potential consumers (at a price) to provide further insights into the donor's character and attributes.

Privileging the Reproduction of 'Biosocial Elites'

Whilst presented by banks as performing a purely facilitative role in gamete selection these devices remain far from innocent. This is because they are employed to hierarchise donors and in so doing to create mechanisms of exclusion for individuals whose 'qualities' or pedigree are deemed to be 'sub-optimal' in husbandry terms. Most US banks actively celebrate this process of discrimination, casting or promoting it in lead banners on their web pages as an assistive tool which helps the consumer to do just that: to discriminate between donors, or, in Callonistic terms, to make evaluative judgements between otherwise similar products. California Cryobank, for example, proudly boasts that they accept less than 1 per cent of all individuals that apply to become donors. Their criteria for inclusion reveal much about why the 'failure' rate is so high. The bank has a formal policy of rejecting any donor who is less than 5 foot 9 inches tall or who is not either currently undertaking a four year degree course at a University or who already has a Bachelor or higher educational degree. They also note that their preference is to 'actively recruit donors from top US universities'.[4] Those who do not conform to these criteria are made to appear as 'outliers' even though, in fact, it is they who make up the largest proportion of the general population. Despite the fact that the individuals that are identified on the basis of this initial social screening already constitute a tiny elite their selection is by no means assured. Rather, the bank considers these qualities to be simply 'basic requirements' for recruitment, noting that only those who meet them will be moved onto 'the next step in our qualification process'. This involves, as they describe it: 'conform[ing] to our unwavering benchmarks by which potential sperm donations are measured, which includes everything from extensive medical testing to genetic screening'.

What is the social programme that is being initiated here, who is initiating it, why and how? Some useful parallels can here be drawn from a comparative analysis of the role of selection in animal breeding programmes. In considering how particular stock comes to be valued and represented much can be gleaned by examining the role of genetic techniques and other calculative devices that are called upon to 'verify' such evaluations and thus rationalise processes of selection and de-selection of donors. As Holloway et al. (2011, p. 533) have recently noted, from the eighteenth century onwards selective breeding has been employed to prosecute the wider political project of agricultural 'improvement' and 'progress'. It involves 'selecting the "best" animals within a population with the aim of producing "better" future generations'. This has historically involved the generation of 'populations level norms against which individuals can be assessed in terms of their conformity or deviation'. These norms, and the hierarchies that they institute, have been formalised through the development of distinctive mechanisms for knowing and evaluating livestock, most notably through the construction and implementation of the concept of pedigree, and scrutiny of pedigree records but also through veterinary checks of animal health. Increasingly however, breeders are now turning to commercial companies who offer analysis

---

4   See details of California Cryobank's donor qualification criteria: <http://www.cryobank.com/How-It-Works/Donor-Qualification/> [Accessed 22 December 2013]. See also <http://www.cryobank.com/uploadedFiles/Cryobankcom/_forms/pdf/brochures/DonorPyramid.pdf>.

of the animal's genetic markers, which as they argue are increasingly being relied upon by breeders to 'sort out "good" from "poor" animals [thereby] producing a clear and actionable hierarchy of animals according to the presence or absence of particular marker genes in their genotype' (Holloway et al., 2011, p. 543).

The question of how to improve 'population quality' through practices of selective reproduction emerged as a key preoccupation not only of agriculturalists but also of demographers through the early decades of the twentieth century. As Frank Dikotter (1998, p. 467) has noted 'far from being a politically conservative and scientifically spurious set of beliefs ... eugenics belonged to the political vocabulary of virtually every significant modernising force between the two world wars including [particularly] in emerging fields such as maternity, psychiatry, criminology, public health and sex education'. Whilst it is often assumed that the eugenicist agenda was fulfilled through the use of radical techniques for curbing the reproduction of those deemed 'unworthy of life' (the retarded or deviant) such as forced sterilisation, its aims were, as Greta Jones (1982, p. 719) reminds us, just as frequently realised through the application of much more subtle interventions. These included, for example, calls to implement national schemes that offered higher rates of family allowance, greater tax deductions and the payment of family bonuses for those in the professional classes; all intentionally designed to 'propagate the fit'. Powered by the prestige of science, eugenics 'allowed modernising elites to represent their prescriptive claims about social order as objective statements grounded irrevocably in the 'laws of nature'; creating in the process a biologising vision of society that 'reduced human life to a hereditary mechanism' (Dikotter, 1998, pp. 468, 476).

It is often assumed that such compulsions and their associated practices become politically indefensible only after the eugenicist programme reached its catastrophic apogee during the Nazi regime. However, whilst its more extreme iterations have mostly been expunged it could be argued that its underlying principles continue to resonate on in equally subtle ways today, and that they are evidenced in the mechanisms of qualification that we see at work in the contemporary marketing of human gametes. Just as in many other domains of production, the product (in this case, donated sperm stored in US banks) is now subjected to an array of testing mechanisms and packaging devices that are called upon to perform the work of establishing its superior quality and in so doing, of singularising it from its competitors. These tests range from those which assess the morphological coherence of the sperm (often determined by reference to masculinist criteria such as its robustness motility and capacity for forward, penetrative movement) but also, increasingly, as in the case with animal breeding programmes, by reference to tests which assess the donor's genetic makeup and social position. Together they are called up to construct what can only be described as a pedigree of the prospective donor – one that consumers are encouraged to employ in making their reproductive selections.

Clear commensurabilities with practices of animal husbandry also emerge here in the modes of classification that are employed to hierarchise donors in the minds of consumers and also in the rationales that they are invited to employ in justifying their right to access these 'superior sires'. The California Cryobank website, for example, promotes a Featured Donor (their iteration of the Bull of The Day) which today is Donor 12977, billed as an 'Athletic and Academic All-Star: a driven charmer ready to take on the world, with two undergraduate degrees and a medical degree in hand. Shy but friendly, this green-eyed overachiever is always looking to challenge himself and excel, whether in the classroom or on the athletic field'. The consumer is not usually asked to take the presence or value of these exceptional qualities on 'face value', rather testing is called upon to 'prove' their existence via the use of metrical technologies (Callon et al., 2002). Here, just as in the world of selective cattle breeding, genetic marker tests are being 'promoted by private companies as a new way to separate out and to define boundaries between desirable and undesirable animals' (Holloway et al., p. 543) but, in so doing, also inevitably create new technologies and devices that actually construct and embed wider societal norms of what counts as 'good' and 'bad' stock – a new set of 'truth claims' about the worth of particular individuals and, moreover, of how that 'worth' might be captured and transmitted both biologically and intergenerationally.

Sarah Franklin (citing Charis Cussins) describes the kinds of 'strategic naturalisation' of particular practices that now occurs in assisted conception which allows, for example, non-traditional means of impregnation – such as conception with donor sperm – to be 'deliberately realigned with more conventional norms of descent through a selective emphasis on some natural facts (such as maternity via pregnancy) rather than others (such as conception via donor)' (Franklin, 2007, p. 202). I would argue that a very similar process of selective naturalisation occurs when practices of selective breeding are more palatably packaged and represented to consumers as simply sensible strategies for maximising healthy outcomes in pregnancy, a tactic that serves to efface the overtly eugenicist philosophy (securing and valorising only donors of 'the highest calibre') that so inflects the discourses and mechanics of donor selection.

Another set of packaging devices employed by US banks draw consumers in with their promise to resolve the perplexing dilemma of how to choose between many possible donors. They do so by appealing to that which the customer already knows and trusts (their own biology) or which has been affirmed societally as being of high value or status (regardless of how tenuous or vacuous these evaluations may prove to be). They do so by offering to find donors who are effectively 'clones' of the consumer, their partner, or A-list Hollywood celebrities. As Sarah Franklin notes, the figure of the clone is deeply troubling to many in advanced Western economies evoking complex anxieties about the loss of individual uniqueness, a fear that what is produced is 'derivative, barren and unoriginal' (2007, p. 203). This horror of unlicensed duplication, she suggests, has 'stigmatized the figure of the double, replicant or multiple', resulting in the prohibition of cloned products [which are] seen as illegitimate 'in the same way that "bastard offspring" are when they are shamed by a lack of proper parentage'. However, the polarity of these dynamics is dramatically reversed here, with the introduction of technologies that invite users to effectively, though not literally, clone either themselves or other desirable individuals. These clones are valued *precisely because* the propriety and the quality of the individuals that they purportedly replicate is, it would seem, already known and assured.

The devices that users are offered to facilitate this kind of 'mini-me' cloning are not designed to endorse or promote difference but rather to assure the replication of standards – in this case to assure the maintenance of the line of what is now described in animal husbandry as 'high genetic merit' individuals and their progeny. Facial recognition software is deployed to recognise and duplicate/mirror the already proven qualities of the recipient or their partner in a donor clone. Users are, in this sense, employing such technologies to judge not only others but inevitably also themselves. The donor clone here acts not to diversify the anticipated progeny but rather to ensure that it remains, as far as possible, a replicant of the parents. A hierarchy of value is thus established in which self-replication trumps dissolution through admixture – a tactic that seemingly confirms the innate superiority of the user's genetic stock.

In an unabashed salute to Victorian physiognomy other applications actually encourage users to take prospective donors 'at face value' by inviting them to make assessments of a donor's character or personality from a momentary reading of their facial features. As Sharrona Pearl (2010, p. 2) has argued physiognomy was embraced in the nineteenth century as it offered 'a way to suture the crisis of urban [modern] interaction by providing a means of making judgements even in the most passing of encounters'. In the equally superficial space of the internet, where interactions remain not simply fleeting but entirely virtual, technologies such as the Bank's 'Celebrity Look Alike' application provide prospective parents with opportunities to arrive at 'quick and dirty judgements' about the similitude of the donor to 'high status' exemplars: the implication presumably being that these facsimiles might prove sufficiently commensurate with the original to act as a satisfactory substitute for them. In so doing they encourage consumers to project their own typologies of value (for example about the value of appearance or likeness to celebrities) onto anonymous donors and to imagine that they will be realised in that individual or their offspring. As an assistive technology for adjudging the worth of donors it leaves something to be desired – after all, what does *looking* like Keanu Reeves actually tell you about *being* like Keanu Reeves? Moreover, those who are 'othered' by such processes of selection are typed as sub-optimal stock and are not made available as 'donor clones'.

That the claims that are made in the name of these forms of 'evaluation' are subject to such little scrutiny bears testament, it would seem, to the success of this normalising project. Let us take the Banks' appeals to pedigree as a case in point. As any clinical geneticist will confirm, the pedigrees that are created from three generational oral family histories do not produce infallible guides to the prevalence or transmission of either particular characteristics or even medical conditions that have a genetic basis. Unlike the extensive genealogical records that are employed to create livestock pedigrees, those generated by sperm banks are produced by interviewing prospective donors about their and their immediate families' medical histories. The accuracy of the information that is proffered by the prospective donor may be compromised by a number of factors. Certain conditions such as mental illness are highly stigmatising and their history within the family may be deliberately obscured over time such that the donor remains unaware of them and thus does not report them. Equally as Wattendorf and Hadley note (2005), other information on medical conditions may not have been shared within the family historically due to cultural or health literacy issues leading to obscuration or misattributions of cause of death. Misassignation of the donor's paternity or maternity (of which they may be unaware) can also discredit the information offered.

The Self-certified Pedigree

The identification of disease clustering from pedigree requires extremely detailed characterisation. Pedigrees that are generated only by reference to information derived from the proband themselves (the individual donor in this case) are the least accurate, being described in Worral et al.'s (2001, p. 1,242) typology as 'unvalidated pedigrees'. Only when triangulated with verifiable information from other extended family members do such pedigrees become 'partially or 'fully' validated. The profound ethical issues that arise from the sharing of medical or genetic information within families (see Lucassen and Parker, 2004) may well prohibit individual donors from providing anything more than a generalised narrative account of what they believe or have been told is their family medical history. The actual utility of such pedigrees remains very limited as they are only self-certified. The genetic tests that are employed to provide the necessary certitude may identify the presence of certain rare single cell conditions but are most likely to identify only probabilistic risk – an increased probability of being affected. Despite this, as Novas and Rose argue (2000, p. 509): 'such individuals may then be treated, by themselves, and by others ranging from employers and insurance companies to future spouses and genetic counsellors, as if their nature and destiny was indelibly "marked" by this genetic flaw. In some cases they may be treated as if they were virtually certain to develop a condition in its most severe form, despite the fact that the "penetrance" of the genes may be unknown, that in most cases only a certain percentage of individuals in this class will suffer in this way, and that the timing of onset and severity of any disorder is unpredictable'.

The presumption that informs these approaches to the marketing of sperm, is, as Wahlberg (2008, p. 191) puts it, that 'quality is *inherent to the biological sample itself* a spurious supposition when determinations of what constitutes 'quality' must of course remain the product of subjective, and as he argues, increasingly 'normative assessments … of what a "good life" or a "life worth living" are'. Focusing so intensively on the quality of the prospective donors is a strategy that invites users to imagine that 'quality control' is therefore assured, neatly obscuring, as it does, that fact that the offspring that results from the use of donor sperm is not cloned but rather a result of 'sexual reproduction and bilateral descent' (Franklin, 2007, p. 202). The pedigree, genetic identity, social standing or morphological quality of the maternal recipient's gametes are not subject to similarly robust regimes of 'product testing' and they may well have a completely countervailing effect on the physical or intellectual development of any offspring conceived from such a union; thereby rendering predictions about the 'quality' of the children produced from these 'premium' gametes unreliable to say the least.

Despite the necessarily imperfect correlation that exists between the 'quality' of the donor and the 'quality' of any child they father, some American banks charge differentially for donor sperm derived from college graduates. Fairfax Cryogenic, for example, hierarchises its fee payments charging 380 US dollars a vial of sperm from anonymous regular donors enrolled in their partner organisation Cryogenic Laboratories, 498 US dollars for their own quality assured Fairfax Graduates 'brand' and 619 US dollars for sperm from Fairfax Graduates who are prepared to be identified to their progeny in later life. Other banks, such as California Cryobank do not levy additional charges to access sperm from more highly educated donors. However, this is somewhat of a red herring given that due to their stringent recruitment regime they *only* accession sperm from such individuals. They do though encourage consumers to believe that ever more finely calibrated information about the donor's biological, genetic and social identity will deliver ever greater degrees of certitude apropos its general superiority. This then provides the necessary justification for triaging access to this information via various levels of paid subscription. At California Cryobank for example, access is ordered via different levels of subscription packages – the first which is free, provides a basic profile, medical history, donor personal essay and staff impression, the Basic at 145 US dollars offers that information and an additional extended donor profile (containing family pedigree and advanced genetic testing); childhood photos and 'express yourself' material; whilst the premium account at 250 US dollars offers all of that and additionally a facial features report, recorded donor conversations and Kiersey behavioural and personality testing. Access to information is thus stratified and paid for differently. A hiearchisation occurs, not just of the donor semen, which is paid for separately, but also of information that 'verifies' the purported quality or character of the material. Consumers are here invited to pay more to access information about pedigree so that they may more easily and assuredly identify 'choice' gametes that can be reserved for their future use. These subscription packages are employed – in Callonistic terms – as a metrical technology for establishing (through objective testing procedures) the value of particular products enabling consumers to singularise their quality in this crowded marketplace.

Conclusion

The emergence of artificial insemination in the seventeenth century and the later refinement of the science of cryogenics together enabled gametes to be mobilised in historically unprecedented ways. With their liberation from the body came new opportunities for them to be circulated and marketed within reproductive economies that are now globally expansive. They also presented new opportunities to place reproductive materials within a competitive market in which the highest economic return was secured only for the 'best' reproductive material that can then be actively employed to prosecute wider political project of population 'improvement'. As I hope I have demonstrated in this chapter, these developments are significant for human sperm banking as they have invoked similar impulses there – providing consumers with new means and opportunities to breed in highly 'selective' ways. However, it is clear that these capacities also usher in new forms of biosociality that that prompt consumers to use risk markers for disease and other metrical tests as helpful tools for identifying 'that sort', 'the ones at risk of having Alzheimer's or an autistic child' (Hacking, 2006, p. 84) despite the fact that we now know that 'everything is *not* in our genes'.

Despite this, the sperm banks and their online interfaces deploy, as I have illustrated here, a sophisticated battery of devices, modes of representation and assistive technologies that would purport to provide their customers with incontestable proof of the genetic merit and pedigree (and thus inherent superiority) of the breed stock they seek to access – one of the factors that undoubtedly serves to make US sperm such a highly desirable export commodity. This is evidenced in the ways in which it is packaged as a product to potential consumers but also in the ways in which those same customers affirm such assertions through their willingness to consume not only the products so marketed but also the attendant narrative about their 'worth'. From this point of view, as Callon, et al. note (2002, p. 201), 'consumers are just as active as the other parties involved. They participate in the process of qualifying available products. It is their ability to judge and evaluate that is mobilized to establish and classify relevant differences'.

Perhaps in the final analysis it is therefore incumbent upon us all to reflect on the role that we as consumers play in the validation of these practices that privilege and seek to perpetuate the reproduction of these new biosocial elites. As Hacking (2006, p. 87) notes, a reasonable fear here is that 'a lust for technology and an admiration for false precision will make genetics override community among not only technocrats but also people in general'. What are our personal responsibilities here – in what ways are all users complicit in constructing such hierarchies and in so doing perpetuating the trope of pedigree with all its implicit value judgements? Whilst these practices of selection are constructed by both customers and banks as constituting sensible strategies for safeguarding a 'better pregnancy' they also simultaneously act to serve the eugenicist agenda of propagating the fit at the expense of those deemed less worthy of reproduction.

Much can be learnt from tracing back the use of artificial insemination and the markets in sperm from their role in animal husbandry and selective breeding to their recent application in the world of human IVF, not least as it serves to highlight that the desire to employ such technologies for population improvement through deselection of defective stock is a compulsion that remains strong to this day. Some caveats can be learnt though from the experiences of the AI industry in cattle where the technology is now much more mature. As Funk has noted (2006, p. 1,367) the AI industry in the US has undergone many consolidations and mergers over the past 25 years such that the industry is now dominated by only five large banks that between them now supply over 90 per cent of US bull semen and which thus dominate the international bull semen export market. The use of a small number of high genetic merit stock to produce this semen has not, however, produced the super breeds that were initially anticipated – instead it has produced worrying high and rapidly increasing rates of in-breeding with associated implications for the quality of stock and their fertility. Consequently industry leaders are now attempting to remedy these defects by instituting 'aggressive programmes to diversify the pedigrees of young sires'.

Whilst there is no possibility that the use of donor sperm will ever account for 95 per cent of human reproduction (although of course that was never anticipated in animal husbandry either) its use is growing within particular constituencies and is evidenced in the burgeoning global market for US donor sperm. Within that market the social construction of some individuals as 'prime' stock has increased demand for their banked gametes such that they also become highly utilised. The absence in the US of binding regulations limiting the number of live births per donor combined with a desire to capitalise on these very highly desirable donations has led US banks to maximise the use of this stock. Consumers also privilege it and it often 'sells out' and has to be reserved in advance. As Pi notes (2009, p. 389), what is 'troublesome is the fact that there are particular characteristics that result in a few frequently requested donors and a bank can divide up a single donation to sell the sperm to numerous recipients such that, as she reveals 'one particular donor, number 1476 of the Fairfax cryobank, is the biological father of at least 36 children born between 2002 and 2007'. Where the recipients are all based in a particular locality this can lead to identified risks of consanguinity. Whilst this is usually the geographic area surrounding a state bank it can also increasingly refer to particular towns or cities internationally that are drawn to the use of particular banks, which, due to similar processes of consolidation to that which have occurred in the AI Cattle industry are now equally small in number.

As Callon, et al. argue (2002, p. 212), as 'the anthropology of consumption has so clearly shown us classifying products, positioning them and evaluating them inevitably leads to the classification of the people attached to those goods'. If we do not want to become an implicit part of the assemblage that so casually calculates the value and worth of the whole of human diversity (finding most sub-optimal or lacking) then it falls to us to carefully reflect on the ways in which we as consumers participate in the processes of evaluation and judgement that underpin not only the definition of the worth of these increasingly valuable commodities but which also clearly drive and shape the cross border economies in gametes in which they are marketed, both nationally and internationally.

References

Almeling, R., 2011. *Sex Cells: The medical market for eggs and sperm*. California: University of California Press.
Barney, S., 2005. Accessing Medicalized Donor Sperm in the US and Britain: An historical narrative. *Sexualities*, 8(2), p. 212.
Bowman, S., 1975. *The Development of Artificial Insemination in Cattle in the United Kingdom*. PhD, University of Cambridge.
Callon, M., Méadel, C. and Rabehariso, V., 2002. The Economy of Qualities. *Economy and Society*, 31(2), pp. 194–217.
Cussins, C., 1996. Ontological Choreography: Agency through objectification in infertility clinics. *Social Studies of Science*, 26(3), pp. 575–610.
Dennison, M., 2007. Revealing Your Sources: The case for non-anonymous gamete donation. *Journal of Life and Health*, 21(1), pp. 15–16.
Dikötter, F., 1998. Race Culture: Recent perspectives on the history of eugenics. *American Historical Review*, 103(2), pp. 467–78.
Edwards, J., Walton, A. and Siebenga, J., 1938. On the Exchange of Bull Semen between England and Holland. *Journal of Agricultural Science*, 28(3), pp. 501–8.
Franklin, S., 1997. *Dolly Mixtures: The remaking of genealogy*. Durham, NC: Duke University Press.
Funk, D., 2006. Major Advances in Globalization and Consolidation of the Artificial Insemination Industry. *Journal of Dairy Science*, 89(4), pp. 1,362–8.
Gürtin, Z. and Inhorn, M., 2011. Introduction: Travelling for conception and the global assisted reproduction market. *Reproductive Biomedicine Online*, 23(5), pp. 535–7.
Hacking, I., 2006. Genetics, Biosocial Groups and the Future of Identity. *Daedalus*, 135(4), pp. 81–95.
Holloway, L., Morris, C., Gilna, B. and D. Gibbs., 2011. Choosing and Rejecting Cattle and Sheep: Changing discourses and practices of (de)selection in pedigree livestock breeding. *Agricultural and Human Values*, 28(4), pp. 533–47.
Jones, G., 1982. Eugenics and Social Policy between the Wars. *The Historical Journal*, 25(3), pp. 717–28.
Lucassen, A. and Parker, M., 2004. Confidentiality and Serious Harm in Genetics: Preserving the confidentiality of one patient and preventing harm to relatives. *European Journal of Human Genetics*, 12(2), pp. 93–7.
Newton-Small, J., 2012. Frozen Assets. *Time*, 16 April, pp. 33–4.
Novas, C. and Rose, N., 2000. Genetic Risk and the Birth of the Somatic Individual. *Economy and Society*, 29(4), pp. 485–513.

Parry, B., 2004. Technologies of Immortality: The brain on ice. *Studies in History and Philosophy of Science Part C: Studies in History and Philosophy of Biological and Biomedical Sciences*, 35(2), pp. 391–413.

Pearl, S., 2010. *About Faces: Physiognomy in nineteenth-century Britain*. Harvard: Harvard University Press.

Pi, L., 2009. Regulating Sperm Donation: Why requiring exposed donation is not the answer. *Duke Journal of Gender Law and Policy*, 16, pp. 379–401.

Pinto-Correia, C., 1997. *The Ovary of Eve*. Chicago: University of Chicago Press.

Rabinow, P., 1992. Artificiality and Enlightenment: From sociobiology to biosociality. In: J. Crary and S. Kwinter, eds. *Incorporations*. New York: Zone Books, ch. 5.

Turkmendag, I. Dingwall, R. and T. Murphy., 2008. The Removal of Donor Anonymity in the UK: Silencing of claims by would-be parents. *International Journal of Law, Policy and the Family*, 22(3), pp. 283–310.

Van Hoof, W. and Pennings, G., 2012. Extraterritorial Laws for Cross-Border Reproductive Care: The issue of legal diversity. *European Journal of Health Law*, 19(2), pp. 187–200.

Wahlberg, A., 2008. Reproductive Medicine and the Concept of 'Quality'. *Clinical Ethics*, 3(4), pp. 189–93.

Wattendorf, D. and Hadley, D., 2005. Family History: The three generation pedigree. *American Family Physician*, 72(3), pp. 441–8.

Worral, B., Chen, D. and Meschia, J., 2001. Ethical and Methodological Issues in Pedigree Stroke Research. *Stroke*, 32(6), pp. 1,242–9.

PART II
Transnational Bio-medical Tourism

Chapter 5

Transnational Health Care: Global Markets and Local Marginalisation in Medical Tourism

John Connell

Introduction

Tourism has long been associated with improved health, by passive relaxation on beaches, more vigorous golf and hiking, and the rise of spas, yoga and rejuvenation treatments: loosely health tourism. Recently a more specific medical tourism has grown with increasing numbers of people travelling across national borders for various treatments, notably cosmetic surgery, dentistry and check-ups, but also for some unusual treatments, such as stem cell surgery, unavailable in home countries. In the past two decades a form of 'reverse globalisation' has brought patients from developed countries to less developed countries for medical care, for a combination of reasons involving cost, access, service and quality. Medical tourism has been said to have grown explosively since the late 1990s with large numbers of patients moving across international borders to countries such as India, Thailand and Mexico in search of medical care usually deemed too expensive at home, or where waiting lists are too long. Since sickness normally induces conservatism rather than expansiveness to a world of opportunities this is a remarkable shift. While contemporary medical tourism is often regarded as having begun in Cuba, it has become a quintessentially capitalist phenomenon and a dynamic example of the transnationalisation of health care, an activity once assumed to be thoroughly local, or at least national, but now globalised.

A formal definition of medical tourism is elusive because of problems of combining intent, procedure and duration, the diverse socio-economic and institutional structures of mobility and disagreements over the nature of 'tourism'. It is probably more useful to conceptualise medical travel as combining all forms of cross border mobility for medical care, avoiding value judgments over intentionality or the gravity and necessity of procedures. Thus medical tourism parallels 'standard' tourism as 'a hybrid economic formation blending different industries, the state, "nature", the informal sector, the capitalist and non-capitalist economies and all manner of technologies, commodities and infrastructures' (Gibson, 2010, p. 529). Growing numbers of countries have enthusiastically marketed themselves as health tourism destinations, hundreds of medical tourism companies have become travel agents, brokering and facilitating medical travel, private hospital chains have extended into medical tourism and across continents and extraordinary claims have been made for the numerical growth of medical tourism, especially by industry participants and destination countries (Connell, 2011a, 2013a). In barely a decade medical tourism has boomed and become highly complex in terms of new destinations, procedures, regulatory regimes, ethics and interlocking entrepreneurialism. Many countries are now involved as both sources and destinations of tourists, as privatisation of medical care continues, discontent with public care increases, cosmetic procedures multiply, baby boom populations age and disposable capital is available. Destination countries seek foreign exchange and new means of economic growth. As technology has improved and diffused and ethical boundaries stretched, the range of procedures has increased and diversity ensued.

Contemporary medical tourism emphasises a number of themes including the privatisation of health care in post-industrial economies, the growing dependence on technology, uneven access to health resources, the accelerated globalisation of both health care and tourism, rampant consumerism and cherishing the body beautiful in an age of entitlement. Despite government promotion and support, medical tourism is emphatically led, and usually exclusively owned, by the private sector, and competition has intensified. In many destinations the development of medical technology and surgical skills, the emergence of a middle class with new needs, privatisation and restructuring after economic problems encouraged supply. In many developing countries, from sub-Saharan Africa to Russia, a growing elite with capital and contempt for local medical care enhanced demand. Its genesis has had few links to health tourism and was entirely pragmatic, resulting in intense competition and a legacy of ethical issues.

Global Intimacy

The most distinctive feature of medical tourism is that it takes patients across international borders, far beyond the perhaps comfortable and familiar cultural relationships sometimes built up over years between health care providers, doctors and patients, to places that may be culturally, climatically and linguistically different and unfamiliar. Crossing such social and political borders for sometimes difficult, unpleasant and intimate procedures, in an unfamiliar and uncertain regulatory environment, can be extremely challenging and accounts for considerable reluctance. Nonetheless patients cross borders to make cost savings, avoid long waiting times and access procedures unavailable at home.

This new international structure and geography of health care provision and mobility has involved building trust with patients, often online and seemingly impersonally, which has been stimulated by the recent rise of medical tourism companies, key elements in marketing. The two most crucial elements in developing contemporary medical tourism have been the rise of the internet, enabling instant access to the web pages of health providers and the rapid growth of medical tourism companies (MTCs), or brokerages, that market medical procedures in distant countries and arrange the linkages between patients and hospitals, travel and accommodation and the tourism that often goes alongside that. The combination of the internet, MTCs and the advice of those who have gone before are crucial influences on the decision-making of medical tourists (Johnston et al., 2012). That in turn has substantially increased the role of social media. Larger MTCs have branches in different countries and with affiliations with hospitals, hotels and airlines. Somewhat scathingly, Turner has described them as 'the car dealerships of the global health-services industry' (2007, p. 127), beyond the bounds of ethics or fiduciary duty, but they are little different from most travel agents.

Linkages between MTCs, hospitals, hotels and airlines emphasises both the privatisation of medical care within medical tourism, the rise of new health conglomerates and the complex transnationalisation of the industry, all exemplified in Asia. New low cost airlines, such as the Malaysia-based AirAsia have actively promoted medical tourism, and many Asian airlines advertise medical tourism in in-flight magazines. Various national airlines have developed special deals for medical tourists. MASholidays, the travel arm of Malaysia Airlines, has incorporated health screening packages into all-inclusive travel packages, targeted at Indonesia, Bangladesh and Vietnam (Connell, 2011a; Anon., 2011a). Lufthansa and Etihad offer similar packages. Like all forms of tourism, marketing the destination and, in the case of medical tourism, marketing specific services in destinations and guaranteeing their quality, is highly important for potential visitors who may be quite unfamiliar with both countries and services, and where patients may only meet 'their medical practitioner' at the moment of the procedure.

Finding a place in an increasingly crowded market is the most basic challenge for countries, corporations and MTCs seeking to develop medical tourism. Many owners of small companies have personal experience and thus personal linkages that sometimes target particularly distinctive groups (Connell, 2011a, p. 95–6). By contrast other MTCs have emerged from wholly commercial considerations as subsidiaries of companies with no links to health. Thus Health and Leisure, which proclaims itself the largest medical tourism facilitator in the Philippines, with various services and links to several providers, emerged from the parent company, Gulf Express Corporation (GEC), which started in the business of airline representation in 1995 and currently holds agreements with some of the most established carriers in the airline industry, including Qantas, Jetstar and Eva Air. It is further linked to travel, construction and engineering companies. Similarly, Elixir Medical Tours was a product of Lotus Forex Limited, a leading Foreign exchange and remittance company based in Hong Kong and with offices in UK, Australia, India, Singapore, Malaysia and Taiwan. The Elixir Medical Tours division started in response to strategic diversification plans, with the intention of 'making forays into the medical tourism sector as Health Travel Facilitators', to promote *medical tourism* in India (quoted in Connell, 2011a, p. 95). Marketing and branding, by MTCs countries, corporations and health care providers are critically important in a highly competitive market, beset by frequent new entries, and where international accreditation, whether formally by JCI or by word of mouth, underpins success.

Privatisation and the New Entrepreneurs

The rise of MTCs is symbolic and symptomatic of the privatisation and marketing of health care. As in Thailand, this rise initially began with the privatisation of health care for more affluent national populations. Thus, Thonburi Hospital in Thailand explicitly 'targets patients with middle class incomes and who prefer the services of a private hospital instead of a public hospital' (Niyomyath, 2009, p. 32). In the wake of the late 1990s Asian financial crisis, which depressed national economies, this middle-class market gradually became an international one (Henderson, 2004; Chee, 2010; Connell, 2011a). Pressure on governments to stimulate economic growth and generate foreign exchange resulted in their supporting, encouraging and marketing medical tourism, and later relaxing regulations and securing accreditation. India, for example, has provided tax incentives, subsidised the industry and created a special visa that doubles the time visitors can stay in the country (up to a year) to receive medical treatment (Chinai and Goswami, 2007). Thailand and Malaysia offer special visas for long-stay health tourists. West Bengal and the Cayman Islands have allocated state land for medical tourism facilities. Since economic liberalisation and deregulation in the mid-1990s two principal private Indian hospital chains, Apollo and Fortis, have expanded and been given government support to import technology and other medical goods with reduced tariffs, so bringing infrastructure in the best hospitals at least to the best western levels.

In their efforts to become the most important global destination, Indian hospitals have upgraded technology, absorbed western medical procedures and protocols and emphasised prompt, low cost attention. Links to India's highly successful IT industry have been advertised as important and symbolic of modernity. Singapore has stressed its ability to successfully implement high-risk procedures, such as the separation of Siamese twins. Ironically, such high-risk procedures are rare in medical tourism where check-ups and other routine procedures such as dentistry dominate (Connell, 2013a). Internationalisation and the marketing of sophisticated procedures necessitated the modernity of technology and health workers. Advertising stressed both, and staff were literally pale reflections of the mass of local health workers, more than evident in casual inspection of websites and advertisements.

The principal corporate hospital chains gradually employed teams of interpreters, though India has benefited because of widespread English speaking ability, especially of those skilled health workers returning from overseas. The Philippines has sought to replicate that success. Mexico has begun to train bilingual English-speaking nurses. Indonesians travel to Malaysia where Malay is comprehensible.

Beyond dominant local and regional mobility, the largest market has long been the Gulf states and several countries have sought to develop strategies to capture that market. Malaysia, notably, has stressed its Islamic credentials, aimed at both the Gulf and Indonesia, and its minority Chinese population, aimed at Singapore and elsewhere, in a deliberate 'strategic cosmopolitanism' (Ormond, 2013a, 2013b). One of the country's leading healthcare providers, KPJ Healthcare, has argued 'It is time for Malaysia to promote the medical tourist sector aggressively to the Arab world' (quoted in Anon., 2012b).

Despite what remains a dominant global image of well-off westerners travelling to distant holiday destinations for often unnecessary cosmetic surgery, medical tourism is dominated by local cross-border movement between neighbouring countries and, in the case of Mexico and India, diaspora populations. Medical tourists primarily seek high-quality care and after care, at reasonable cost without waiting times and in an accessible and reasonably comfortable and congenial context. Several countries, notably India, have developed their medical tourism industry on the basis of encouraging the return of diaspora populations. Mexicali, on the United States border, has constructed a special border crossing lane, to give priority to medical tourists (Anon., 2012c). Jordan aims at a broad Arabian diaspora. Other countries seeking to enter the industry, such as the Philippines and Jamaica, have focused marketing efforts on diaspora populations and stressing the cultural benefits: HealthCore Philippines, a local MTC, argues that, 'It is better for Filipinos abroad to get healthcare procedures in the Philippines because they have relatives here and they are familiar with the language' (quoted in Anon., 2011b). That perspective has drawn diaspora populations to Taiwan (despite competition with Singapore) and Korea. Yet the 'holy grail' of medical tourism remains gaining access to the affluent United States market.

Liberalisation and privatisation brought new structures of corporatisation that, in India, streamlined the notorious bureaucracy and significantly improved administration. Especially in Asia many leading private hospitals, where medical tourism is significant, are part of international chains; typified by Parkway Holdings (Parkway Pantai Limited), the main Singapore hospital chain, with its flagship Mount Elizabeth hospital, which by the mid-2000s had become a regional conglomerate. Parkway Holdings owned and managed hospitals, dental surgeries, diagnostic labs and research facilities in several Asian countries alongside being engaged in the sale of properties, and investment holding and trading activities. In 2005, when it claimed that 40 per cent of its income came from foreign patients, it had marketing offices in 15 countries, including Indonesia, Malaysia, China, India, Bangladesh, Sri Lanka, Vietnam, Brunei, UAE, UK, Russia and Canada (Khalik, 2006). Five years later it had been briefly taken over by the Indian based Fortis Healthcare, only to be subsequently sold to Khazanah, the state investment company of Malaysia. Khazanah also has a 12.5 per cent share in the Indian Apollo hospital chain. By 2012 Parkway was the second largest health care provider in Malaysia (where it had 11 hospitals with three more under construction) and had some clinical or hospital presence in China, Hong Kong, India Vietnam and Brunei, with planned expansion into Indonesia, Sri Lanka, Turkey and elsewhere. It also owns and manages general, dental and radiology clinics, deals in medical supplies, owns a clinical research centre and provides diagnostic laboratory services. Its 2010 Annual Report proclaimed it to be 'Asia's leading private healthcare player, with a strong brand, unparalleled geographical network and a value proposition [*sic*] that is renowned globally' (Parkway Holdings Limited, 2011, p. 3).

Fortis Healthcare, a large New Delhi based chain with a dozen large sophisticated hospitals, was set up by Ranbaxy Laboratories, the largest drug company in India. It owns Wockhardt and other smaller hospital groups, including the Escorts chain. Its purchase of a stake in Parkway early in 2010, significantly expanded its scale of operations and its overseas linkages to a total of over 62 hospitals, as it became the largest hospital network in Asia. After acquiring the major shareholding in Parkway, in 2010, Fortis's Chairman explained:

> The next phase of our growth will be well beyond Asia. Our ambition is to strengthen our brand at a global level. First step in this strategy was to penetrate the Indian market, which we have done through Fortis Healthcare and Fortis Hospitals. The next step is to establish a footprint in Asia … done through our acquisition of Parkway. Parkway's strong presence in Malaysia with the Pantai group gives us great confidence. This gives us a strong platform to leverage our partnership to position ourselves for the next phase of growth outside Asia. This acquisition will significantly expand our footprint across the region and place us strategically and geographically for geographical and clinical leadership in Asia, a big step close to our vision of establishing a global healthcare delivery network. (quoted in Connell, 2011a, p. xx)

In this drive for global expansion the role and content of health care itself was scarcely prominent. By 2012 Fortis Healthcare had 75 hospitals in eleven countries. Its website stated: 'The healthcare verticals of the company span diagnostics, primary care, day care specialty and hospitals, with an asset base in 11 countries, many of which represent the fastest-growing healthcare delivery markets in the world' (fortishealthcare.com2012).

International linkages and investments constantly change, reflecting the intricacies of ownership and intense competition, and complicating the marketing of medical tourism in terms of the balance between Asian countries, including the 'big four' of Thailand, India, Singapore and Malaysia, and the efforts of others to break in. India can compete most effectively on price but Singapore competes on technical ability (quality) and cleanliness, hence there is scope for some complementarity. That became evident in 2010 when the major Indian hospital operator Fortis Healthcare purchased a substantial share in Singapore's Parkway Holdings, Parkway having a reputation as one of Singapore's best hospital groups. Transborder institutional linages and differences are increasingly subtle:

Indian hospitals are generally much less expensive than those in Singapore or other medical-tourism destinations such as Thailand or the Philippines. For instance, a hip replacement that costs $43,000 in the US could cost $12,000 in Singapore and just $9,000 in India. Convincing Americans to jet off to third-world India is a bit of a harder sell, though. By buying a 23.9 per cent stake in Parkway from US private equity firm TPG for $687 million, Fortis has now positioned itself to become the regional leader in medical tourism, with a strong presence in India (where it has 46 hospitals) for the most price-sensitive patients and a new base in Singapore for higher-end customers aiming for more luxury (Einhorn, 2010).

Medical tourism has here contributed to internationalisation, new relationships between countries, new forms of private sector investment and the emergence and growth of 'classical' but new transnational corporations. For instance, the Apollo Group, the largest group based in India and sometimes claimed to be the world's third largest private health provider, is involved in multiple health care related activities, ranging from provision of regional telemedicine services from centres in south and south-east Asia, to provision of back-office services to US organisations for billing, documentation of administrative records and coding of medical processes and insurance claims. It has 50 hospitals across Asia, including Sri Lanka and Bangladesh, and smaller faculties in Ghana, Nigeria and Mauritius, and it has agreed to move into Tanzania.

Hospitals have also become more transnational with links between hospitals in the Global North and South as investment becomes more important. Just as the United States hospital chain Johns Hopkins has branches in Singapore and Dubai, so numerous Asian hospitals claim affiliations with hospitals in the United States. Fortis and Apollo have formed partnerships with Johns Hopkins Medicine International and the Wockhardt Group, initially a mainly pharmaceutical and diagnostics company, is affiliated with Harvard Medical International, who manage some 25 hospitals across India (Medhekar, 2011). While hospitals themselves have become transnational they have partly done so by becoming part of much larger conglomerates, many of which take in more than only the health and travel industries. Groups such as Apollo, Fortis and Parkway dominate the medical tourism industry in India and Singapore.

Health care is increasingly integrated with other economic activities as in Thailand where airlines have a substantial stake in medical tourism. Bangkok Airways, Thailand's largest privately owned airline, has built 'wellness centres' for medical tourism, and owns three Bangkok hospitals. The national airline, Thai International, like Malaysia's MAS, has packages including medical check-ups as part of its Royal Orchid Holidays. Patients at several Bangkok hospitals can obtain frequent flier points for their treatment costs. Bumrungrad and the Bangkok Hospital Group have welcoming booths and concierge services at Bangkok Airport. One of the largest Thai cosmetic surgeries has opened branches in Dubai and Vietnam. Bumrungrad International Hospital, the most prominent hospital engaged in medical tourism (whose website claims patients from 190 countries) has a majority 56 per cent stake in Manila's newest private medical centre, Asian Hospital, another in Dubai, a renal centre in Singapore and manages two other international hospitals in Yangon, Myanmar and Dhaka, Bangladesh.

Once distinct industries and corporations are increasingly integrated institutionally and across borders. Thus, Bumrungrad International Limited, for example, has clinics and hospitals in eight countries. In addition to 16 clinics in Thailand, 32 were in Taiwan, 22 in Singapore, 12 in the Philippines, 10 in Korea, 8 in Malaysia and 2 in Japan. From 2007 to 2011 it had a management agreement with Abu Dhabi to operate the Al Mafraq hospital a 500-bed public hospital that treats 310,000 patients a year. By contrast, in 2011 it sold off its Singapore-based subsidiary Asia Renal Care, a kidney dialysis provider with numerous clinics throughout Asia, including Taiwan, Japan, Korea, Malaysia and the Philippines, and purchased the local Kasemrad Hospital Group. Bumrungrad's strategic partners are Istithmar, the investment arm of the UAE government, Temasek (the equivalent in Singapore) Asia Financial Holdings in Hong Kong and the Bangkok Bank. These strategic partners 'are internationally well known with strong presence in their respective regions, thereby providing important sources of new investment opportunities and referral networks especially in the Middle East and Asia' (Bumrungrad Hospital Limited, 2010, p. 58). While referrals may be important the strategic partnerships emphasise that Bumrungrad is simply a private corporation with an interest in profitability. By 2011 Bumrungrad claimed 400,000 international patients, not all medical tourists (Connell, 2011a), and this 40 per cent of all patients contributed about 63 per cent of its income.

Similar aspirations towards a more global presence are evident elsewhere. Indian investments have entered the wealthy Caribbean territory of the Cayman Islands (Connell, 2013b), Taiwanese interests intend to build a world-class Chinese language hospital at Subic Bay in the Philippines to attract a mainland Chinese market, and the Formosa Plastics Group owns a major hotel in Xiamen, China (Reisman, 2010). Each illustrates how hospital chains seek to move closer to markets. Apollo had 37 hospitals in India in 2004, partnerships in hospitals in Kuwait, Sri Lanka and Nigeria, and plans for others in Dubai, Bangladesh, Pakistan, Tanzania, Ghana, Singapore, Philippines, London and Chicago as privatised corporations grew and international linkages intensified. Not all these plans eventuated, and those in Pakistan, London and Chicago were still to eventuate, though Apollo had grown to owning 53 hospitals by 2012.

International investment in medical tourism has become geographically strategic, with transnational medical corporations in many regions making similar decisions to ensure market access close to the source of patients, partly represented in several contemporary developments in the Caribbean (Connell, 2011a, 2013b). In 2010 the Indian hospital chain Narayana Hrudayalaya (NH) signed a joint venture with the Cayman Islands government to build a Health City, eventually to have a 2,000-bed teaching hospital, staffed by Indian specialists. That placed it on the border of the American market. NH, based in Bangalore, has 14 hospitals in India, with major equity investors including JP Morgan and the global insurer American International Group (AIG). The Cayman Islands Health City was intended to be a prototype and blueprint for initially extending the NH chain beyond India and subsequently creating a hospital chain across Africa, where building and management costs are lower, human resources are cheaper and there is greater flexibility and fewer regulations since 'the governments are desperate' (Anon., 2012a).

Hospital executives move between sectors and industries, and in magazines like *Medical Tourism Magazine* excel in the language of business and management efficiency, regularly quoting business gurus such as Peter Drucker, in a world of clients and consumers rather than patients. The executive summary of Bumrungrad's 2009 Annual Report stated that it was 'aggressively looking for additional healthcare opportunities in the region' while its CEO noted that it 'continues to find ways to leverage its brand and intellectual property to open future business opportunities' (Bumrungrad Hospital Limited, 2010, p. 56). Puerto Rico's recent attempts to develop medical tourism have been associated with government tax incentives that have also enabled health service providers 'to become more aggressive' (Connell, 2013b). The Director of NH, Dr Devi Shetty, has described the company's approach to 'cost-effective' patient care as being 'the "WalMart-ization" of medicine – making quality health care more accessible and affordable, through its doctors working longer hours and performing more surgeries than American doctors' (Doyle, 2012). He has also said that he sought to apply Henry Ford's philosophy towards the Indian health care system using mass production techniques to cut costs through specialisation and economies of scale (Anon., 2012a).

While conglomerates in Asia are extending to developed countries, health care providers in developed countries have expanded outwards in more familiar circumstances. Early in 2010, for example, the Harley Street Fertility Centre merged with the London Fertility Centre to concentrate its British operations with the founder of the centre moving to Mauritius to expand development there, rather than in the United Kingdom. As the former reported:

> During his absences from UK, Mr Goswamy has been at his Fertility Centre in Mauritius, building research, teaching and treatment facilities to help many more couples worldwide, especially those who cannot afford to have treatment in London. Many couples have benefited from this two pronged approach to help them achieve their goal of a healthy and happy family. (harleystreetfertility. com, 2012)

Ensuring a stake in a distant market demands some degree of mobility, flexibility, competiveness and globalisation. Thus, just as Bumrungrad has invested in a private hospital in Dubai to move closer to the Gulf market, so some United States dentists, recognising the challenge of Mexican competition, have set up branches of their own businesses there to take advantage of lower costs. The Dallas-based International Hospital Corporation is building and operating hospitals in Mexico that meet American standards. This gradual 'multinationalisation' of health businesses reflects very similar, but more long-established, practices in the tourism industry and also in the manufacturing sector, as companies seek to escape what amounts to local protectionism and tariff barriers. Medical tourism has not just been one component of the globalisation of the health care industry it has actively encouraged and directed it.

Tourism by Default?

Healthcare transnationals are partly integrated with the wider tourism and transport sectors. This is most evident in advertising. India's long established *Incredible India* theme, Thailand's *Amazing Thailand* and Malaysia's *Malaysia Truly Asia* have each included medical tourism, with the industries further benefiting from government investment and subsidy. Being a tourist destination may be conducive to medical tourism and recuperation. Most Bangkok hospitals offer and organise night markets and nightclub shows and sightseeing.

Modernity, in a medical and cultural context, is a drawcard. The redesign of the atrium of Bumrungrad to include Starbucks and McDonalds 'had a powerful effect on lower-income and middle-income Americans [who] discovered that they could afford posh "VIP" services reserved for only the wealthiest clients at private American hospitals' (Turner, 2007a, p. 116). Having Starbucks and McDonald's investing in the hospital offered independent prestige, and accreditation, for visitors from many countries and enables others to have accessible food without stepping outside their comfort zone. In the Gulf, Eastern Europe and other parts of Asia such outlets are symbols of modernity.

As Bumrungrad has expanded its corporate presence outside Thailand, and Thai doctors have migrated to better paid opportunities in those places, Bumrungrad itself, with Starbucks, McDonalds and Au Bon Pain in the foyer, has minimal Asian ambience (more closely resembling a corporate global office or hotel). Its small food court, and the flower shop and newsagents hint at a small shopping mall, an example of what has been described elsewhere as the 'malling of medicine' (Kearns and Gesler, 1998). A travel agency and a visa centre on the third floor organise travel, tours, theatre and concert visits for patients and their relatives. An enthusiastic American health tourist was moved to report that: 'the hospital looks quite modern and even the faint hospital smell is masked by an overriding odor of capitalism' (Leenhouts, 2009, p. 23).

The hospitals at the core of medical tourism have transformed themselves, from the dowdy, functional and clinical public hospitals that preceded them. In the late twentieth century, hospitals went from being functional, technological places to more open human landscapes and living spaces (Sternberg, 2009). Corporate hospitals took on elements of elite hotels, IT offices and shopping malls with an architecture that projects 'the corporate hospital as anything but a hospital' (Lefebvre, 2008, p. 102). Hospitals in Costa Rica have IMAX cinemas and helicopter landing pads. Samitivej in Bangkok offers free wireless internet access to all international patients. Bangkok Hospital provides cable television with various language channels, microwave ovens and guest sofa-beds. The newest projects such as the Indian hotel chain Welcomgroup's Fortune Park Lake City hotel, claims to be a hotel within a hospital, being on the grounds of the Jupiter Lifeline Hospital in Mumbai, and part owned by the hospital: a prototype 'hospitel'. In form and function leading hospitals in the medical tourism industry have come close to luxury hotels, in a transition where consumption and consumerism have been added to cure and care; thus, more like the basic elements of an international tourism industry. A degree of convergence has occurred, hospitals have become less daunting and functional and nearby hotels more oriented to the needs of medical tourism. Some have even seen the emerging linkages between hotels and hospitals, and to nearby places of consumption, as a shift towards 'health theme parks' (Lefebvre, 2008).

Some hospital chains have become functionally integrated into the tourist industry. Bumrungrad owns 74 serviced apartments and 54 hospitality suites, for patients and families, with a swimming pool and fitness facilities. The principal hospital group in Singapore, Raffles, arranges airport transfers, books relatives into hotels and helps arrange local tours. Indian hospitals have similarly become integrated into a wider network. Upmarket private hospitals offer airport pickups and packages that include surgery and several nights' accommodation at high quality hotels. Hotels in Malaysia have similarly become horizontally integrated with hospitals. Costa Rica has specialised in 'recovery retreats', hotel or ranch-style accommodation – a 'hybrid of hotel, home and clinic' exclusively for recovering patients and close to their hospitals, with the amenities of standard hotels but also staffed by nurses and interns (Ackerman, 2010). While tourism may not be the defining element of medical tourism, it both contributes to the tourist industry and is even linked in to it. In most cases it involves various elements of standard tourism. While it can be considered one specialised niche in the tourist industry common usage of the term rarely considers recreation let alone hedonism.

Ethics and Inequality

While the economic benefits from medical tourism have proved elusive to quantification they are nonetheless considerable and account for both the enthusiasm of many countries to participate and growing attempts by many source countries, notably Nigeria and several Gulf states, to discourage mobility, improve local facilities, services and cost regimes and retain patients. In some circumstances economic benefits have seemingly overwhelmed ethical considerations, especially in the poorest countries, anxious to establish a seemingly profitable venture but not easily able to compete in terms of cost and quality. Political and economic factors have also influenced and stimulated the privatisation of medical care and the concentration of financial and human resources in this sector, perhaps to the disadvantage of other sectors and some geographical regions.

Medical tourism has raised complex ethical questions, in terms of the acceptability of particular forms of medical treatment and through broader questions about the impact of medical tourism on local access to health care. That is not surprising: medical practice in any form is open to more ethical considerations than most forms of welfare and service provision. Most ethical debates over medical tourism have centred on certain specific procedures, such as the pathologising of (usually) women's body shapes, surrogacy and the 'fertility industry', 'anchor babies', abortions, organ transplants and stem cell therapy, some being regarded as 'rogue medical tourism' (Hunter and Oultram, 2010; Inhorn et al., 2012), and discussed elsewhere in this book. However, medical tourism has also raised equally complex questions about the appropriate use of skilled health workers and the allocation of financial resources, and, therefore, concerns over social justice and health equity in destinations where health care is presently limited and human resources are stretched.

Medical tourism raises both ethical and practical questions over the appropriate use of medical resources at different scales, whether hospitals or skilled health workers, when such resources are in short supply and thus whether it distorts national health priorities at the expense of private gains. An orientation towards foreigners, who can afford to pay, perhaps at the expense of local people who cannot, parallels the rise of exotic spa resorts, oriented to a luxury market and requiring local obsequiousness, raising similar questions about tourism, ethics and inequality. Thus it has been argued that 'a dual medical system has emerged in which specialization in cardiology, opthalmology and plastic surgery serves the foreign and wealthy domestic patients while the local populations lack basics such as sanitation, clean water and regular deworming' (Bookman and Bookman, 2007, p. 7). Medical tourism draws away resources that might otherwise benefit the public health system (Vijaya, 2010). While Indian private sector hospitals argue that private payments for medical care, and hotels and other services, will trickle down and benefit the economy as a whole, there is little real evidence of this in the absence of effective taxation policies (Chinai and Goswami, 2007, p. 165). Medical tourism has therefore been characterised as a 'form of neocolonialism' (Buzinde and Yarnal, 2012).

Several hospitals in India have been built to meet the needs of medical tourists. Though a growing trend, most hospitals with a significant medical tourism orientation, such as Bumrungrad, remain dominated by national patients. International patients rarely make up even 10 per cent of most hospitals' patients, and in Singapore less than 3 per cent (Chee, 2011). A general outcome of medical tourism has been the more rapid rise of a private health sector labour market in medical tourism destinations, as the economic benefits from employment in that sector become greater, with the consequent movement of health workers into the urban, private sector (Spitzer, 2009), sometimes from rural and regional areas. Such migration has exacerbated existing regional inequalities in access to health care.

Attractive private sector opportunities, now increased through medical tourism, have been a significant influence on migration (Connell, 2010), intensifying national imbalances in health care provision. For example, a substantial part of the disease burden in India is related to infectious diseases such as malaria and tuberculosis.

However, these receive only limited focus and have no relationship to medical tourism, and states where such diseases flourish, such as Bihar and Uttar Pradesh, are highly disadvantaged. Further, urban bias in health care delivery has intensified everywhere. In Malaysia health care delivery is increasingly inequitable (Rasiah et al., 2009). And in Thailand there is a huge drain on the public health sector. To practise medicine in Thailand you must pass a Thai language examination, so the booming private sector can take staff from only one place. Hence, as the secretary general of the Thai Holistic Health Foundation has pointed out, 'In the past we had a brain drain; doctors wanted to work outside the country to make more money. Now they don't have to leave the country, the brain drain is another part of our own society' (quoted in Connell, 2011a, p. 149).

With significant sectoral income differentials doctors have moved into private sector hospitals as part of an 'internal brain drain' where, even by 2003, 'providing health services for foreign patients creates heavy investment in advanced health technology for the private sector at the expense of public health. This enhances the existing tiered health care system, with shifting of human resources for health from the rural public to the urban privates services, resulting in increasing inequity' where 'the resources needed to provide services to one foreigner may be equivalent to those used to provide service to 4–5 Thais' (Wibulpolprasert et al., 2004, p. 5). A Thai doctor observed in 2006: 'Each time a foreigner sees a Thai doctor at 'foreigner prices' he takes away an opportunity for a Thai person to see the same doctor at normal Thai fees. In other words, this programme, while presumably bringing foreign capital to our hospitals, is sucking medical care from our own people' (quoted in Cohen, 2008, p. 250). Medical tourism has resulted in a 'brain drain of medical specialists' including doctors, nurses and pharmacists, from top public hospitals and medical schools, though some of these have returned from overseas (Poopat, 2010; Kanchanachitra et al., 2011). The flow of doctors into the urban private sector is accentuated by foreign preferences for experienced and skilled doctors (NaRanong and NaRanong, 2011), while few doctors wish to be involved in regional primary and preventive health care (Whittaker, 2008).

Growing national support for medical tourism, through more active promotion, land provision, tax concessions on technology purchase, supportive employment tax regimes, et cetera, may simultaneously weaken support for and reduce resources allocated to public health and primary health care. In Thailand and Malaysia powerful interest groups have driven the expansion of the private sector in tandem with medical tourism, with the government subsequently stimulating the expansion of medical tourism in the drive for new market access (Rasiah et al., 2009). The same broad combination of privatisation, large conglomerates and government nurture, with a steady rise in private sector expenditure on health services, has occurred throughout Asia, with similar outcomes, including: greater specialisation in the private sector, limited preventive health care provision and the slow immiserisation of the public sector.

Competition is rife at different scales. In Thailand, for example, 'the private healthcare industry is a fragmented market and only a few hospitals are operating close to their full capacity [hence] the competition for patients remains intense' (Bumrungrad Hospital Limited, 2010, p. 60), at a time when queues in public hospitals are lengthy and parts of the country poorly served. The best metropolitan hospitals, where medical tourism is a part of their activities, have drawn skilled resources away from regional areas and smaller hospitals as part of a continued process combining privatisation, urban bias and the weakening and withdrawal of national planning.

As more and more countries seek to become medical tourism destinations, competition has engendered something of a 'race to the bottom'. Present trends to extend medical tourism to the Caribbean, for example, constitute a move into a region already characterised as being one where outmigration of skilled health workers has left poorer states especially with considerably fewer workers, especially nurses, than are required for adequate and effective care (Connell, 2007, 2010). Diversion of more such workers to providing services for non-residents, while generating revenue, is likely to worsen existing access to health care for the relatively poor, as it has done elsewhere (Connell, 2011b).

While privatisation has raised standards of care and contributed to the improvement of medical facilities in many countries, notably India and Thailand, the most prestigious hospitals are scarcely accessible to most nationals and technological and other benefits have failed to trickle down structurally or geographically to where they are most needed. However an emerging duality may not be entirely rigid, and in regimes of privatisation such groups would be marginalised and ignored in any case, as they have so often previously been. Medical tourism has emphasised this and made disparities more acute and more visible, especially in areas such as reproductive tourism, stem cell surgery (and adoption) where costs are very high and only mobile elites benefit, but it is not the main cause of health worker shortages and maldistribution.

The rise of medical tourism has coincided with the ascent of neo-liberalism, the privatisation of hospital facilities and declining or static investment in the private sector. Ultimately 'the neo-liberal paradigm of cost-effective and consumer-friendly private markets falls short of consumer welfare and public good' (Cook et al., 2013, p. 69; Smith, 2012). While privatisation has raised standards of care and contributed to the improvement of medical facilities in many countries, the most prestigious hospitals are inaccessible to most nationals, and technological and financial benefits have failed to trickle down, structurally or geographically, while skilled labour has gravitated upwards. Medical tourism has reinforced privatisation and contributed to these trends.

Conclusion

Medical tourism is the latest phase of a continuously expanding diversity of therapeutic places, from the biomedicine of Harley Street and the thousands of formal health care facilities, big and small, through landscapes and places of 'natural' and 'traditional' remedies to the expanding medical tourist destinations of Asia, Latin America and Central Europe. New rivals constantly appear. China is a very slowly emerging player. The growth of medical tourism has given a dramatic emphasis to the internationalisation of medical services, and the remarkable globalisation of practices and procedures once regarded as fundamentally intimate, but now subordinated to the logic of an international market (Parry, 2008). While the industry touts public–private partnerships (Medhekar, 2011), governments are usually not much more than facilitators, reducing bureaucracy, promoting a positive vision of the country and developing legislation. Medical tourism has reinforced privatisation alongside a technological and medicalised view of the health system where medical services can be bought 'off the shelf' from the lowest cost provider, rather than wellbeing created by remedying the social, political and economic determinants of health: an analogy with the relationship between cosmetic surgery and diet and exercise.

Greater expectations, rising affluence, media depictions of what is appropriate and normal have fuelled searches, made feasible by the internet and the subsequent rise of MTCs, and aggressive marketing, for alternatives to slow and narrow local, public choices and perspectives. Medical tourists have been seen to be moving away from the sometimes rigid constraints of national health care systems and their perceived inadequacies. Insurance companies are also opting to send patients overseas to reduce their own costs (Connell, 2011a). Japanese companies send employees to Thailand and Singapore for annual physical examinations, as the savings on medical fees and high quality medical care make the air fares and accommodation costs inconsequential. New international institutional structures have emerged.

The incursions of capitalism and commodification into hitherto personal and private experiences, from birth through to death, that are suggestive of a materialist, egoistical and self-absorbed society, are symptomatic of much of medical tourism, which has both stimulated and responded to such trends. It reduces pressures on governments, as the more affluent and powerful move in or move out. The private medicine that is epitomised in the principle centres of medical tourism offers examples of places and providers that are not only sites of treatment but key elements in emerging and highly competitive neo-liberal landscapes of discretionary consumption (Kearns et al., 2003), where advertising and marketing play a critical role, and links with international companies, from Starbucks to Flight Centre, are as significant as those with pharmaceutical companies.

Globalisation manifestly offers new opportunities and greater mobility, new flows in a compressed world, yet at the same time it enhances structural inequalities, that tend to empower those who are relatively well off at the expense of the less privileged, so that globalisation is far from a uniform process. The globalisation of the market for medical treatment parallels both the now global market for skilled health care workers (Connell, 2010), the universal privatisation of health care and the emergence of global insurance companies. This has been matched by the individualisation of patients who have an unprecedented freedom to choose (and outsource themselves) as long as they also have a capacity to pay.

A global shortage of specialists and professionals, including doctors, pharmacists and technicians, has slowed growth, while political problems, high costs, poor infrastructure, remoteness, language differences and unfamiliarity have prevented significant growth beyond the principal early innovators. Only exceptionally do the relatively poor become medical tourists. Likewise, markets are rather more regional than global. Hospital chains too are regional, analogous to older TNCs and integrated with them. Thus medical tourism comes ever closer to representing 'the full integration of medicine with global capitalism' and, where service is purely a function of the ability to pay, redeeming features are elusive in a system that tolerates 'striking inequalities in income and health' (Turner, 2007, pp. 113, 128; cf. Cohen, 2011). There is little evidence that it has attracted beneficial foreign investment, except perhaps in parts of the tourist industry, that competition has benefited the health sector as a whole, that greater numbers of skilled health workers have been produced, or corporate social responsibility increased, even on the part of the more successful hospitals. In this perspective medical tourism is both symbol and manifestation of the failures of both privatisation and of public national health care systems.

Yet, inside and outside the 'neo-liberal landscapes' of corporate wellbeing, patients have been obvious beneficiaries, some moving away from difficult local circumstances (such as many of those from Mexico and Yemen), waiting lists and spiralling costs, and gaining healthy new lives (even perhaps at the expense of some national citizens). However inadequately measured, or simply ignored, medical tourism has also contributed to employment. As in almost every tourism context, large companies (the MTCs, the travel industry and also the providers) are the main beneficiaries, the tourists get more or less what they anticipate and have paid for and the local population (including such direct providers as surrogate mothers and liver donors) are least likely to experience trickledown effects. In this emerging nexus of complex privatisations, links with components of the tourism industry provide institutional evidence that medical procedures overseas are not merely of clinical interest, but that they constitute a distinct niche in the tourism industry.

Hospitals have become interlocking conglomerates, extending into health education, clinical research, medical technology, IT and beyond that into the tourist industry. Property and insurance companies have moved into hospital ownership and medical tourism. The flattening world of biotechnology incorporates supply chains of sperm (directed by internet orders), pharmaceutical supply chains, the globalisation of surgery via robotics and telemedicine, global diagnostic radiology, web-surfing for providers and the expanding global franchises (of hospitals, hotels and MTCs) with large medical conglomerates. Medical tourism enhances these trends and is likely to increase further in future as medical care continues to be increasingly funded by overseas investment, technology improves in developing countries, word of mouth extends, public sector healthcare is underfunded, populations age, expectations increase and significant cost differentials remain. It will be an increasingly competitive and aggressive business, at some odds with the tourist imagery.

References

Ackerman, S., 2010. Plastic Paradise: Transforming bodies and selves in Costa Rica's cosmetic surgery tourism industry. *Medical Anthropology*, 29(4), pp. 403–23.

Anon., 2011a. Partnership with Airline to Boost Medical Tourism. *International Medical Travel Journal*, 22 September.

———, 2011b. Overseas Filipinos Become Key Target for Philippine Medical Tourism. *International Medical Travel Journal*, 14 November.

———, 2012a. Medical Tourism Developments in the Caribbean. *International Medical Travel Journal*, 7 September.

———, 2012b. Malaysian Medical Tourism on the Increase. *International Medical Travel Journal*, 4 October.

———, 2012c. Mexico Increases Efforts to Attract US Medical Tourists. *International Medical Travel Journal*, 18 May.

Bookman, M. and Bookman, K., 2007. *Medical Tourism in Developing Countries*. Basingstoke: Palgrave Macmillan.

Bumrungrad Hospital Limited., 2010. *Annual Report 2009*. Bangkok.

Buzinde, C. and Yarnal, C., 2012. Therapeutic Landscapes and Postcolonial Theory: A theoretical approach to medical tourism. *Social Science and Medicine*, 74(5), pp. 783–7.

Chee, H.L., 2010. Medical Tourism and the State in Malaysia and Singapore. *Global Social Policy*, 10(3), pp. 336–57.

Chinai, R. and Goswami, R., 2007. Medical Visas Mark Growth of Indian Medical Tourism. *Bulletin of the World Health Organisation*, 85(3), pp. 164–5.

Cohen, E., 2008. Medical Tourism in Thailand. In: E. Cohen, ed. 2008. *Explorations in Thai Tourism*. Bingley: Emerald, pp. 225–55.

Cohen, G., 2011. Medical Tourism, Access to Health Care, and Global Justice. *Virginia Journal of International Law*, 52. [online] Available at: <http://heinonline.org/HOL/Page?handle=hein.journals/vajint52&div=4&g_sent=1&collection=journals> [Accessed 18 July 2013].

Connell, J., 2007. Local Skills and Global Markets? The migration of health workers from Caribbean and Pacific island states. *Social and Economic Studies*, 56, pp. 67–95.

———, 2010. *Migration and the Globalisation of Health Care*. London: Edward Elgar.

———, 2011a. *Medical Tourism*. Wallingford: CABI.

———, 2011b. A New Inequality? Privatisation, urban bias, migration and medical tourism. *Asia Pacific Viewpoint*, 52(3), pp. 260–71.

————, 2013a. Contemporary Medical Tourism: Conceptualisation, culture and commodification. *Tourism Management*, 34, pp. 1–13.

————, 2013b. Medical Tourism in the Caribbean Islands. A cure for economies in crisis? *Island Studies Journal*, 8(1), pp. 115–30.

Cook, P., Kendall, G., Michael, M. and Brown, N., 2013. Medical Tourism, Xenotourism and Client Expectations. Between bioscience and responsibilisation. In: C.M. Hall, ed. 2013. *Medical Tourism. The ethics, regulation and marketing of health mobility*. London and New York: Routledge, pp. 61–74.

Doyle, J., 2012. Ascension Health Plans $2 Billion Cayman 'Health City' Project. *Medical Tourism Magazine Newsletter*, 1 May.

Einhorn, B., 2010. India Company's Medical-Tourism Push. *Bloomberg Business Week*. [online] Available at: <http://blogs.businessweek.com/mt/mt-tb.cgi/16544.1387312592> [Accessed 12 March 2013].

Fortis Health Care, 2012. Saving and Enriching lives [online]. Available at:<http://www.fortishealthcare.com > [Accessed 12 September 2012].

Gibson, C., 2010. Geographies of Tourism: (Un)ethical encounters. *Progress in Human Geography*, 34(4), pp. 521–7.

Harley Street Fertility Centre, 2012. Harley Street Fertility Centre [online] Available at: http://www.harleystreetfertility.com> [Accessed 25 August 2012].

Henderson, J., 2004. Healthcare in Southeast Asia. *Tourism Review International*, 7, pp. 111–22.

Hunter, D. and Oultram, S., 2010. The Ethical and Policy Implications of Rogue Medical Tourism. *Global Social Policy*, 10(3), pp. 297–9.

Inhorn, M., Shrivastav, P. and Ptrizio, P., 2012. Assisted Reproductive Technologies and Fertility 'Tourism': Examples from global Dubai and the Ivy League. *Medical Anthropology*, 31(3), pp. 249–65.

Johnston, R., Crooks, V. and Snyder, J., 2012. 'I Didn't Even Know What I Was Looking For'. A qualitative study of the decision-making processes of Canadian medical tourists. *Globalization and Health*, 8. [online] Available at: < http://www.globalizationandhealth.com/content/8/1/23> [Accessed 18 July 2013].

Kanchanachitra, C., Lindelow, M., Johnston, T., Hanvoravongchai, P., Lorenzo, M. et al., 2011. Human Resources for Health in Southeast Asia: Shortages, distributional challenges, and international trade in health services. *The Lancet*, 377(9,767), pp. 769–81.

Kearns, R., Barnett, J. and Newman, D., 2003. Placing Private Health Care: Reading Ascot hospital in the landscape of contemporary Auckland. *Social Science and Medicine*, 56(11), pp. 2,303–15.

Kearns, R. and Gesler, W., 1998. *Putting Health Into Place*. New York: Syracuse University Press.

Khalik, S., 2006. Foreigners Flocking to Singapore Hospitals. *The Straits Times*, 29 March, pp. 1–2.

Leenhouts, P., 2009. Thank Goodness for Ladyboys. My (brief) experience with medical tourism, *Medica Tourism*, 1, pp. 23–4.

Lefebvre, B., 2008. The Indian Corporate Hospitals: Touching middle class lives. In: C. Jaffelot and P. van de Veer, eds. 2008. *Patterns of Middle Class Consumption in India and China*. New Delhi: Sage, pp. 88–109.

Medhekar, A., 2011. Public-Private Partnerships for Sustainable Growth of Medical Tourism. *Medical Tourism Magazine*, 21, pp. 51–4.

NaRanong, A. and NaRanong, V., 2011. The Effects of Medical Tourism: Thailand's experience. *Bulletin of the World Health Organisation*, 89(5), pp. 336–44.

Niyomyath, W., 2009. Bone Therapy. *Medica Tourism*, 1, pp. 31–3.

Ormond, M., 2013a. Claiming 'Cultural Competence'. The promotion of multi-ethnic Malaysia as a medical tourism destination. In: C.M. Hall, ed. 2013. *Medical Tourism. The ethics, regulation and marketing of health mobility*. London and New York: Routledge, pp. 187–200.

———, 2013b. *International Medical Travel and the Politics of Therapeutic Place-Making in Malaysia*. London and New York: Routledge.

Parkway Holdings Limited, 2011. *2010 Report Card*. Singapore.

Parry, B., 2008. Entangled Exchange: Reconceptualising the characterisation and practice of bodily commodification. *Geoforum*, 39(3), pp. 1,133–44.

Poopta, T., 2010. Earning Tourist Dollars without Trauma. *The Nation* (Bangkok), 2 November, 10A.

Rasiah, R., Noh, A. and Tumin, M., 2009. Privatising Healthcare in Malaysia: Power, policy and profits. *Journal of Contemporary Asia*, 39(1), pp. 50–62.

Reisman, D., 2010. *Health Tourism. Social welfare through international trade*. Cheltenham: Edward Elgar.

Smith, K., 2012. The Problematization of Medical Tourism: A critique of neoliberalism. *Developing World Bioethics*, 12(1), pp. 1–8.

Spitzer, D., 2009. Ayurvedic Tourism in Kerala: Local identities and global markets. In: T. Winter, P. Teo and T. Chang, eds. 2009. *Asia on Tour. Exploring the rise of Asian tourism*. Abingdon: Routledge, pp. 138–50.

Sternberg, E., 2009. *Healing Spaces*. Cambridge, MA: Belknap Press.

Turner, L., 2007. From Durham to Delhi: 'Medical tourism' and the global economy. In: J. Cohen-Kohler and M. Seaton, eds. 2007. *Comparative Program on Health and Society*. Lupina Foundation Working Paper Series 2006–2007, University of Toronto, pp. 109–31.

Vijaya, R., 2010. Medical Tourism: Revenue generation or international transfer of healthcare problems? *Journal of Economic Issues*, 44(1), pp. 53–70.

Whittaker, A., 2008. Pleasure and Pain: Medical travel in Asia. *Global Public Health*, 3(3), pp. 271–90.

Wibulpolprasert, S., Pachanee, C., Pitayarangsarit, S. and Hempisut, P., 2004. International Service Trade and its Implications for Human Resources for Health: A case study of Thailand. *Human Resources for Health*, 2(10), pp. 1–12.

Chapter 6

Bioethics, Transnational Health Care and the Global Marketplace in Health Services

Leigh Turner

Introduction

Health-related travel, often labelled 'medical tourism', involves intranational and transnational movement for the purpose of obtaining medical care. Though many countries arrange state-facilitated and publicly-funded cross-border health care, medical tourism typically involves individually planned medical care that is purchased as an out-of-pocket expense. Medical tourism is a contested concept and the phrase is used in many different ways. Acknowledging the plurality of manners in which this phrase is used, otherwise diverse contributors to ethical, social and economic analysis of the subject agree that medical tourism refers to the practice of individuals who intentionally travel for the purpose of obtaining desired medical interventions. The phrase does not encompass business travel, holiday travel or other instances in which individuals travel to a region beyond their country of residence and then, with no prior plans for seeking medical treatment abroad, require health care following injury or illness.

Despite extensive news media coverage and considerable scholarly research documenting the expansion of medical tourism, there is little reliable evidence concerning how many patients cross national borders for the purpose of obtaining health care (Lunt and Carrera, 2010). Recognising the need for more accurate counts of transnational flows of patients, it appears that increasing numbers of patients are leaving their home countries and arranging health care in nations marketing themselves as destination sites for medical tourists. Popular destination countries for medical tourists include the Czech Republic, Hungary, Poland and Ukraine in Eastern Europe; Mexico and the United States in North America; Argentina, Brazil and Venezuela in South America; Barbados, Cuba, Dominican Republic, Jamaica and Puerto Rico in the Caribbean; and India, Indonesia, Malaysia, Singapore, South Korea, Thailand and the Philippines in Asia (Connell, 2006). India is particularly well-known as a country advertising inexpensive health care but it is important to emphasise that many nations are now attempting to build 'bioeconomies' and promote themselves as attractive destinations for medical travellers. Though transnational medical travel is often described using the popular label medical tourism, there is risk in associating the word *tourism* with the provision of health services. The label could trivialise what often are consequential journeys involving serious medical procedures. The phrases *transnational health care* and *international medical travel* are sometimes used as alternate labels because of the association of the word tourism with relaxation and pleasure-seeking, recreational travel and holiday excursions (Kangas, 2002).

Reasons for Transnational Medical Travel

There are many reasons why patients seek health care outside the countries in which they reside (Arellano, 2007). Some patients lack health insurance or are underinsured (Milstein and Smith, 2006). This problem is particularly acute in the United States (Milstein and Smith, 2007). Some uninsured Americans seek inexpensive health care in such countries as Mexico and India because they are not covered by public health insurance plans or private health insurance and they cannot afford the cost of care at US medical facilities (Mitka, 2009). Other patients travel for care even though they live in countries with publicly funded health insurance plans and they do not face medical debt or health-related bankruptcy if they obtain care at local medical facilities. Wait times in Canada, for example, result in some patients paying out-of-pocket and obtaining prompt access to care in foreign countries rather than waiting for publicly funded treatment in their communities (Eggertson, 2006). Some individuals seek access to medical interventions that are illegal in their home communities. For example, some patients suffering from renal failure travel to Egypt, India, Pakistan or the Philippines and purchase kidneys from impoverished, desperate individuals (Scheper-Hughes, 2003). Other patients undergo medical procedures that are not approved in their home nations. Some individuals with multiple sclerosis, amyotrophic lateral sclerosis, Parkinson's disease and other serious illnesses travel to such countries as India, Thailand, Mexico and the Ukraine and seek 'stem cell' interventions that have not been tested in clinical trials or received regulatory approval (Kiatpongsan and Sipp, 2009). Little is known about the safety, effectiveness and risk-benefit ratio of these procedures. Some individuals journey to assisted reproduction clinics and arrange sex selection, commercial surrogacy and other practices that are prohibited in their home nations (Inhorn and Patrizio, 2009). Other patients seek medical care at international facilities because of limited access to health care in their home nations (Kangas, 2002). Some patients fly to India, Mexico or elsewhere because they are immigrants and they prefer arranging health care back in their communities of origin (Lee, Kearns and Friesen, 2010; Bergmark, Barr and Garcia, 2010). Finally, though this cohort of patients receives only limited scrutiny in scholarship examining transnational medical travel, some patients obtain access to alternative healing practices or indigenous forms of medicine that are unavailable in their local communities. In short, there are numerous reasons why patients arrange health care at international hospitals and clinics. Cost gradients matter but affordability of care is not the only reason why patients enter the global marketplace in health services.

Organisations Promoting Medical Tourism

Many organisations are involved in the establishment of a global marketplace in health services. Medical tourism companies are proliferating in countries to which patients travel for care, nations from which patients depart for treatment and in third-party countries that are neither departure points nor destinations for medical travellers (Lunt, Hardey and Mannion, 2010). Medical tourism facilitators commonly market a 'basket' of medical procedures, provide 'price bands' or 'price points', build networks of international health care providers and advertise side trips, hotel accommodations and travel arrangements for customers. Just as medical tourism companies seek to expand their client base, hospitals and clinics in many different nations use marketing strategies to attract international patients. Joint Commission International and other accreditation bodies play an important role in promoting the understanding that select medical facilities provide 'international' standards of care (Crone, 2008). Perhaps most importantly, regional and national governments in India, Malaysia, Singapore, Thailand and many other countries promote medical tourism initiatives as a means of attracting travellers, boosting revenues from tourism and increasing foreign direct investment (Bennet, 2007).

Many business enterprises, government agencies and other organisations are attempting to promote expansion of transnational patient travel. Despite various sources of support for the development of a global marketplace in health services, there are numerous unresolved ethical, legal, clinical and public health issues associated with the medical tourism industry. These topics deserve careful consideration even though in some instances the current evidence base is too limited to make definitive judgments about social benefits and harms related to transnational medical travel. Proponents of a globalised marketplace in health services highlight the benefits of medical travel. Acknowledging that there are circumstances where travel in search of health care is beneficial, it is also important to identify risks and harms associated with transnational medical travel and the emergence of a global healthcare marketplace.

Profit-maximising Strategies and Best Interests of Patients

Little is known about how medical tourism companies and destination health care facilities market procedures to medical tourists. It is conceivable that framing effects driven by commercial interests have a powerful influence upon how risks and benefits for particular procedures are described to medical tourists. Medical tourism companies, destination hospitals and participating health care providers all profit when patients decide to travel and purchase health services. The more health care packages patients agree to purchase, the more various parties profit from these economic transactions.

In settings around the world, fee-for-service payment of health care providers raises concerns that medically unnecessary interventions are provided as a revenue-generating strategy. Financial conflicts-of-interest are evident in the medical tourism industry, but they can be found wherever health care facilities and providers can maximise financial gain by increasing the volume of diagnostic tests and clinical procedures. Practice guidelines, notions of medical professionalism, fiduciary obligations, legal concepts such as medical negligence and personal injury and ethical norms such as avoiding doing harm and promoting the best interests of the patient are supposed to provide normative channels that prevent caregivers from being guided by pure profit-seeking. Medical care is supposed to be 'evidence-based' rather than driven by financial interests of health care providers. However, in the global health care marketplace, where regulatory standards are variable and different understandings of professionalism and accountability are present, some patients might be at risk of undergoing medical procedures that are not medically necessary. Two publications examining episodes of transnational medical travel describe circumstances in which patients were advised by their local physicians to pursue conservative, non-surgical forms of addressing health problems (Cheung and Wilson, 2007; Walker, Brooker and Gelman, 2009). In both instances, the patients went abroad, arranged care at international medical facilities and returned home with serious complications. One patient had a gynaecological procedure in India and the second patient had a knee replacement in Thailand. Clinicians can, of course, disagree over effective means of addressing health problems. Furthermore, there might be some benefits associated with the emergence of a 'medical consumerist' ethos that limits the capacity of local health care providers to act as gatekeepers to health services sought by patients. Noting these caveats, it is important to state that one significant danger associated with the development of a global marketplace in health services is that medical tourism companies and destination hospitals might sometimes sell medical procedures that are not in the best interests of patients. The fusion of transnational medical travel with medical consumerism and a highly commercialised, privatised form of medical care could result in provision of health services that profit health care providers but offer limited benefits to patients and in other instances put patients at considerable risk of harm.

Informed and Uninformed Consent

At present, there are no 'microsocial' studies investigating conversations medical travellers have with agents, facilitators or brokers working for medical tourism companies as well as the international patient departments of destination hospitals. When patients from such countries as Australia, Canada, England and the United States seek treatment in their home countries, health care providers are bound by professional standards, institutional policies, case law and legislation concerning information disclosure, patient decision-making capacity and informed patient choice. Before patients decide whether to provide consent to particular interventions there are legal and ethical norms in place that are supposed to ensure that they are provided information concerning risks and benefits of undergoing procedures, treatment alternatives and their risks and benefits and risks and benefits associated with declining recommended interventions. Legislation governing patient–physician communication, information disclosure and informed consent processes varies across legal jurisdictions, but the general purpose of such legislation is to ensure that patients are provided with the information they require to comprehend and weigh treatment-related risks and make informed choices. Patients must be able to interpret and understand the information they are given, comprehend the consequences that can flow from their decisions and have decision-making capacity. Though social practices of information disclosure and patient decision-making are culturally situated, over the last four decades many countries around the world have attempted to improve patient access to information and ensure that patients are given opportunities to make informed choices before deciding whether to undergo particular medical interventions. In previous decades medical parentalism was regarded as a major barrier to informed patient choices. In the current era, economic interests of health care providers might serve as a significant impediment to informed patient decision-making.

One noteworthy ethical issue associated with globalisation of health services is that marketing of medical tourism could involve exaggerating benefits and minimising risks associated with undergoing medical procedures. Medical tourism companies typically receive payment for referring patients to destination hospitals or earn a percentage of fees charged to their clients. Sellers of health services do not receive financial rewards for encouraging non-interventionist or inexpensive preventive approaches to management of health problems. Rather, they profit when clients purchase health services. It is conceivable that powerful financial incentives shape exchanges among medical travellers and representatives of medical tourism companies and destination hospitals. If economic incentives shape how information is provided, it is plausible that in some instances where health services are marketed, risks are minimised, benefits are exaggerated and patients are not given all the information needed to help them make informed decisions. When travelling abroad for care, many patients might experience a significant gap between the information they would receive were they to arrange care at health care facilities in their local community and the information they are provided by medical tourism company representatives and clinicians at destination hospitals (Lunt, Hardey and Mannion, 2010). Future studies by medical anthropologists, medical sociologists and other social scientists likely will examine specific social and clinical encounters in which health services are marketed to transnational medical travellers. Even prior to publication of such studies there are legitimate grounds for concern about how economic incentives might influence how risks and benefits of care are described to transnational medical travellers.

Continuity of Care

A significant ethical and clinical problem associated with arranging health care at international medical facilities is that continuity of care can be compromised. Geographically dispersed medical care, even with the emergence of various forms of telemedicine, can be fragmented and episodic. Medical tourism is often marketed as providing prompt access to inexpensive surgical procedures. However, the need for competent care extends beyond time in the operating room. Patients need and must have opportunities to consult with health care providers before undergoing medical procedures. Likewise, post-operative care and long-term follow-up care needs to be arranged when patients undergo surgery. In general, surgeons either continue to see their patients following surgery or transfer care of their patients to other clinicians. Failure to arrange suitable post-operative care is in many jurisdictions a serious breach of the fiduciary obligations of clinicians.

A growing body of scholarship and news media coverage indicates that some medical travellers return home without adequate plans for post-operative health care (Furuya, Paez, Srinivasan et al., 2008; Hanna et al., 2009; Newman, Camberos and Ascherman, 2005). Some medical travellers return home without pre-existing arrangements for post-surgical monitoring and treatment, and only receive medical attention after being taken to emergency rooms (Yang et al., 2009; Reed, 2008). Continuity of care is a serious challenge when patients obtain medical care far from where their family doctor or general practitioner is located (Turner, 2007b). Continuity of care for medical travellers is further compromised by the reluctance of some physicians to provide care after a patient has gone abroad and undergone surgery in a distant country. Some clinicians worry that they will become targets of litigation if they attempt to address health problems of patients who have received care elsewhere. International teleradiology, videoconferencing, instant messaging and other forms of telecommunication provide technical means for promoting communication between health care providers located in different countries (Wachter, 2006). Nonetheless, numerous factors contribute to fragmented care when medical travellers arrange treatment abroad. The importance of continuity of care in treating illnesses and injuries raises significant questions about the ethics of encouraging large numbers of patients to enter a global health services marketplace and obtain health care in distant settings.

Privacy and Confidentiality of Medical Records

There is little reliable information concerning privacy of patient data and confidentiality of medical records when patients cross borders in search of health care. Though medical tourism companies play a role in organising patient travel, these businesses are not medical clinics or hospitals. It is unclear how well they preserve confidentiality of medical information. At present, no studies examine how medical records and other forms of personal information are transmitted electronically by medical tourism companies to destination health care facilities. With regard to destination hospitals and clinics, there is presumably considerable variation in how effectively particular medical facilities protect privacy and confidentiality of patient information. Recognising the limited evidence available to address this topic, websites of destination hospitals and medical tourism companies suggest that transnational medical care sometimes involves activities that do little to protect privacy of patient information and confidentiality of medical records. Some medical tourism companies and destination hospitals identify patients by name, disclose the procedures they underwent and provide typically confidential information such as private mobile phone numbers and town or city of residence.

Inadequate Infection Control and Surgical Technique

There are no systematic, comprehensive studies revealing how many medical travellers suffer from post-surgical infections and substandard surgical techniques. Systematic assessment of clinical outcomes in transnational medical travel would provide insight into whether patients are at greater risk of harm when they travel abroad for care. Though there are no comparative studies examining clinical outcomes in transnational medical travel, there are numerous case reports of patients returning home after receiving care abroad and having to undergo revision surgery, treatment for infections that are likely a result of inadequate sterilisation and infection control measures and other forms of care (Birch et al., 2010; Birch, Caulfield and Ramakrishnan, 2007; Jeevan and Armstrong, 2008). These studies cannot be used to make categorical, sweeping claims about quality of care at international medical facilities. Definitive judgments about quality of care in transnational medical travel would first require a better understanding of how many patients cross borders for care and how many travellers experience substandard care at particular destinations. Recognising the need for detailed comparative studies of quality of care and patient safety in different health systems, case reports published to date generate questions about quality of care at specific hospitals and clinics. Some patients return home and require costly follow-up care. International health care providers typically do not play a role in treating these post-surgical health problems. In addition, they often do not assume financial or legal responsibility for post-operative care required following hospital-acquired infection or what in communities in which medical tourists reside would be classified as medically negligent care (Burkett, 2007; Cortez, 2010; Mirrer-Singer, 2007). Given that many patients leave medical tourism destinations shortly after receiving care, it is possible that clinicians at international health care facilities are unaware of most instances in which medical travellers require extensive follow-up care after their return home. This failure to track outcomes data is a marked departure from standard tracking of surgical outcomes data.

In countries around the world, and in health care systems within countries, there can be significant variations in the professional capabilities of health care providers, standards for licensure, infection control in operating rooms and wards, quality of blood supply and screening of tissues and organs, quality of medical devices and surgical equipment and integrity and quality of medications (Green, 2008; Farrugia, 2009). Some medical travellers presumably journey to health care facilities offering high-quality professional care. Other patients risk encountering institutions and clinicians with lower standards for clinical practice and patient care. Hospital acquired infections and substandard medical procedures can both lead to increased rates of morbidity and mortality.

Surgery, Air Travel, and Thrombotic Events

To limit travel costs, some medical travellers schedule brief stays at medical tourism destinations and fly home shortly after having surgery. Patients who travel shortly before or after surgery and who are not treated prophylactically before beginning long-haul flights are at increased risk of deep vein thrombosis and pulmonary embolisms (Handschin, Banic and Constantinescu, 2007; Bhatia et al., 2009; Feltracco et al., 2007). In brief, combining surgery and long-distance air travel puts patients at increased risk of blood clots. These clots can lead to a range of outcomes extending from mild discomfort to death. Although there is an extensive body of research addressing 'economy-class syndrome', few articles examine deep vein thrombosis and pulmonary embolisms in medical travellers. There are no epidemiological studies that attempt to quantify for transnational health care travellers risks associated with flying long distances days before or after surgery. In addition, contemporary health research does not address whether international medical facilities and medical tourism companies provide medical travellers with detailed information concerning risks associated with air travel shortly before and after surgery. Given the risk of deep vein thrombosis, pulmonary embolism, post-surgical infections and other complications following medical interventions, there is reason to speculate about the period of time during which medical travellers should avoid flying following surgery. Focusing upon economic advantages of travelling to inexpensive health care facilities might result in insufficient attention being paid to risks associated with deliberately combining surgery with long distance flights. The very notion of combining long-distance travel with surgical procedures deserves critical analysis. Many transnational medical travellers are likely being subjected to risks of which they are unaware. Because blood clots can occur after surgery even without long-distance air travel, detailed epidemiological studies are needed to better understand the extent to which combining surgery with air travel increases patients' risks of thrombotic events and pulmonary embolisms. Since medical travellers start their journeys at different points and travel to many different destinations, there are numerous practical obstacles to conducting systematic studies examining the consequences of taking long-haul flights shortly after surgery.

'Bargain-Priced' Care and Costs to Publicly Funded Health Care Systems

Cost of care is an important consideration for many patients as they decide whether and where to travel for treatment. Though quality of care presumably matters to medical travellers, one prevalent marketing strategy of destination health care facilities is to promote inexpensive procedures (Turner, 2007a). While individuals should be free to cross national borders for medical care or other reasons, it is important to understand that individual decisions to seek international medical care can have significant collective costs when patients return to their home countries and require care provided by publicly funded health care systems. If growing numbers of medical travellers return home with complications and require costly treatment, it will become increasingly important to recognise transnational medical care as not just a personal choice but also as an activity having significant implications for publicly funded health care systems in nations to which patients return after receiving care abroad. Individual decisions to arrange 'affordable' health care at international sites can impose substantial costs on publicly funded health care facilities in the communities to which medical tourists return after receiving treatment abroad.

There is considerable disagreement concerning whether publicly funded health insurance plans should cover cost of treating complications after patients have travelled to international health care destinations and then returned home. Health care providers in both Australia and England question whether public health insurance plans should have to cover all health care costs resulting from individual decisions to seek inexpensive medical care abroad (Cheung and Wilson, 2007; Jeevan and Armstrong, 2008). If such episodes become more commonplace, some publicly funded health insurance plans likely will refuse to cover cost of care required following treatment abroad.

Lack of Legal Remedies

Some individuals travel abroad, receive satisfactory care and then return home without experiencing infections or complications. Any attempt to address ethical dimensions of transnational medical travel needs to acknowledge that some travellers receive safe, effective and beneficial medical care. However, for those patients who receive substandard medical care, legal remedies are often unavailable (Burkett, 2007; Cortez, 2010; Mirrer-Singer, 2007; Svantesson, 2008). When individuals purchase health services through medical tourism companies, customers typically sign waiver of liability forms. These documents state that the medical tourism company assumes no liability in the event the patient is harmed while receiving care. Waivers of liability typically indicate that clients of medical tourism companies must sue hospitals and health care providers in the countries within which health care providers are located. These documents are intended to serve as shields by protecting medical tourism companies from lawsuits.

Medical tourism companies' routine use of waiver of liability documents raises serious ethical and legal concerns because many medical travellers will find it difficult to obtain legal redress in the leading destinations for medical tourism. There are numerous obstacles to suing for medical negligence or personal injury in the legal systems of such countries as India, Thailand and Mexico (Cortez, 2008; Cortez, 2010). First, medical tourists must arrange legal representation in the country where they obtained medical care. Second, they must find a court willing to hear the claim. Third, in many countries, legal proceedings will occur in a language that is other than the language spoken by the traveller. Fourth, in many nations there is little likelihood that the patient's case will be heard in a timely manner. Fifth, in some countries establishing medical negligence is very difficult. Some nations are notorious for offering few legal remedies for victims of medical negligence. Sixth, financial settlements in countries where patients travel for medical care are typically paltry in comparison to settlements reached in countries from which many medical tourists originate. Finally, even if a medical tourist wins a judgment, collecting a settlement can prove impossible. Travellers to international medical facilities need to understand that they might find themselves unable to obtain compensation in their home country and in the nation where they received treatment.

Lack of legal recourse for medical tourists might have a dampening effect upon willingness to travel abroad for care. Another possibility is that countries positioning themselves as destinations for medical tourism will reform existing legal frameworks and offer improved mechanisms for pursuing legal action when patients seek redress after being harmed while receiving care (Cortez, 2009). A third option is that insurance companies will devise new insurance products for transnational medical travellers. A final potential scenario is that transnational medical travel will continue to expand because patients do not appreciate the lack of access they will have to legal remedies if they experience negligent medical care and are harmed while receiving treatment at international hospitals and clinics.

Harms to Public Health in Destination Nations

In addition to identifying and examining risks to which individual travellers are exposed, it is important to note that transnational medical travel can harm public health in destination nations (Hazarika, 2009; Sen Gupta, 2008). There are several respects in which promoting medical tourism could have deleterious effects in such countries as India, Thailand, Indonesia and the Philippines. National and regional efforts to build medical tourism infrastructure can result in public funds being used to construct elite facilities catering to wealthy local individuals and international patients. Using government resources to support construction of 'five star' hospitals for international patients can result in 'perverse subsidies' for medical travellers and insufficient resources for improving local population health (Thomas and Krishnan, 2010).

Promoting medical travel risks exacerbating health inequalities. Rather than addressing needs of the most vulnerable members of society and promoting health equity, efforts to promote medical tourism can further polarise already highly stratified societies (Hazarika, 2009; Chaudhuri, 2008; Garud, 2005). 'Trickle down' economic benefits can be limited. Elite medical facilities are often inaccessible to local populations. In countries where organ trafficking occurs, an influx of international patients can result in impoverished local citizens being used as a biological resource for comparatively wealthy individuals (Scheper-Hughes, 2000). Numerous studies document the harmful clinical, social, psychological and economic consequences that result when impoverished individuals attempt to extricate themselves from debt by selling a kidney to international buyers (Padilla, 2009; Scheper-Hughes, 2000; Moazam, Zaman, Jafarey, 2009).

The establishment of elite biomedical facilities in highly stratified economic and social orders can have a dramatic effect upon the capacity to staff public health care facilities. There is a risk that doctors and nurses will migrate from public hospitals to private hospitals, and shift from publicly funded health care systems to the provision of private, for-profit medicine targeted at patients who can afford to pay for care. Promotion of medical tourism as national economic initiative risks increasing rather than decreasing health inequalities.

An influx of medical travellers can also have harmful effects upon the practice of medicine. Health care providers operating in a highly competitive, profit-driven environment can find themselves 'incentivised' to offer the most lucrative tests and therapies rather than providing interventions most likely to improve population health or the wellbeing of individual patients. Promotion of medical travel can also result in purchase of expensive diagnostic equipment and medical devices that benefit medical travellers but are unaffordable and therefore inaccessible to most local citizens. The practical outcome of regional and national efforts to promote medical tourism can be a health care system in which advanced biomedical technologies are available to wealthy consumers while basic medical interventions are withheld from individuals unable to pay for treatment. The public health consequences of a surge in the number of medical tourists travelling to particular destinations are not fully understood, but it is far from obvious that efforts to promote medical tourism in India, Thailand, the Philippines and elsewhere have had meaningful economic, social and public health benefits for local populations. Medical tourism initiatives risk undermining health equity.

Transnational Medical Travel, Infectious Diseases, and Antibiotic Resistance

In addition to posing risks to public health in destination nations, transnational medical travel also generates risks to public health in home countries of medical tourists (Harling et al., 2007). When medical travellers journey abroad for health care and then return with transplanted organs or tissues that have been inadequately tested and screened, or acquire infectious diseases from blood transfusions or inadequate infection control during surgery, they are at risk of spreading infectious diseases in their home communities. These infectious diseases can spread to family members and friends, the larger community and to health care providers and other patients if medical travellers require hospitalisation and medical care upon their return home. In addition, medical travellers who obtain health care at international facilities with high rates of antibiotic resistant infections are at risk for bringing these antibiotic resistant diseases home with them (Krishna, 2010; Muir and Weinbren, 2010; Kumarasamy et al., 2010). These infections are notoriously difficult to treat because standard antibiotic regimens are ineffective against them. Effective infection control measures can reduce the spread of antibiotic resistant infections but isolating and treating medical tourists with diseases resistant to most standard antibiotics will likely prove costly to publicly funded health care systems. The transnational spread of antibiotic resistant infections is likely to receive intense scrutiny in future research on the clinical, public health, and economic implications of medical tourism.

Cross-Border Health Insurance Fraud

Proponents of a global marketplace in health services promote cross-border portability of health insurance (Mattoo and Rathindran, 2006). They recommend expanding networks of health care providers to include foreign hospitals and clinics meeting international accreditation standards. They argue that customers can be offered comparatively inexpensive health insurance plans if they agree to undergo specified elective medical procedures at designated international facilities. It is possible to permit transnational health insurance claims to be made when health care is obtained in international contexts with high standards of professionalism, auditing mechanisms and functioning tools for identifying fraudulent claims. However, supporters of the globalisation of health services and portability of health insurance need to acknowledge the risk of transnational health insurance fraud. In the United States, from the 1990s to the present, the Federal Bureau of Investigation has launched three major investigations of fraudulent health insurance claims submitted when Americans with US health insurance plans visited clinics and hospitals in Mexico (Kranhold, 1997; O'Connor, 1997; Shroder, 2009). In some instances US citizens colluded with health care providers in Mexico, obtained elective cosmetic surgery procedures and then made fraudulent claims for coverage of 'emergency' medical procedures. In other instances, US citizens with minor health problems visited facilities in Mexico and then discovered that the hospitals and clinics submitted inflated claims to US-based health insurers. Efforts to make health insurance globally 'portable' need to recognise the risk of cross-border health insurance fraud. It is possible that the risk of international health insurance fraud is so great that health insurance for cross-border health-related travel will need to be limited to defined areas such as the European Union and will not become truly global in scope. Cross-border investigations of health fraud are complicated, costly and time-consuming and law enforcement agencies often have difficulty disrupting health insurance fraud when fraudulent behaviour occurs in countries outside their usual area of jurisdiction. Though there are various strategies for investigating and prosecuting cross-border health insurance fraud, it is important to recognise the basic point that globalisation of health care likely will be accompanied by globalisation of health insurance fraud.

Organ Trafficking and Exploitation of Vulnerable Populations

One form of transnational medical travel is particularly noteworthy for the harms it inflicts on citizens of such countries as Egypt, India, Pakistan and the Philippines. Organ trafficking, sometimes referred to as 'transplant tourism', involves travel of individuals from comparatively wealthy nations to low-income nations with high levels of poverty and corruption. In these settings, kidneys are available for purchase in black market settings. These operations pose risks to purchasers of commercial organ transplants. Inadequate testing and screening of organs can lead to transmission of infectious diseases from organ sellers to transplant recipients. Several studies document morbidity and mortality in purchasers of commercially acquired kidneys (Yakupoglu et al., 2009; Geddes et al., 2008; Higgins et al., 2003). Sellers of kidneys are also harmed by these transactions. Social scientists and health researchers document how kidney selling can lead to isolation and stigmatisation, diminished health status, surgical complications, infections and other harmful outcomes (Budiani-Saberi and Delmonico, 2008; Delmonico, 2009). Proponents of markets for kidneys claim that when impoverished individuals sell a kidney they can use earnings from these transactions to improve their financial circumstances and extricate themselves from poverty (Radcliffe-Richards et al., 1998). Studies conducted in many different social and cultural settings reveal that kidney selling does not help individuals escape from poverty and debt. Rather, kidney selling often leads to worsened health status and reduced financial resources for sellers and family members. Many kidney sellers become unable to perform demanding physical labour after surgery. Furthermore, debt collectors often demand the money sellers receive for their kidneys. In short, the argument that kidney selling serves as an effective poverty alleviation strategy is unpersuasive and unsupported by available evidence.

It is important to note that buying and selling of kidneys at international health care facilities in such countries as Pakistan and the Philippines generates ethical concerns that do not extend to all forms of health-related travel. Transnational organ trafficking generates significant harms to impoverished individuals in low-income nations. These persons are exploited, their organs are commoditised and commercialised and poor individuals are used as a living biological resource by medical travellers from such comparatively wealthy nations as Australia, Canada, the United Kingdom and the United States. This topic is the subject of detailed critical analysis in numerous publications. Here it is important to note how this particular form of medical travel poses serious risks to citizens living in conditions of poverty.

Conclusion

Hospitals and clinics seeking to attract international patients, medical tourism companies, government agencies and other organisations all promote transnational medical travel. Many businesses see economic opportunities in increasing the number of patients travelling for health services. Regional and national governments regard medical tourism as a means to boost tourism, attract foreign direct investment, and build health care infrastructure (Turner, 2007a; Whittaker, 2008). Advocates of medical tourism use sophisticated marketing strategies to promote globalisation of health care. Notwithstanding claims about the advantages of a global marketplace in health services, there are many grounds for reservations about efforts to 'globalise' patient care. Standards governing information disclosure and informed consent, privacy and confidentiality of medical records, screening of blood products and tissues, medical education and professional licensure, surgical technique and infection control and medical professionalism are highly variable around the world. Though international accreditation bodies exist, quality of care is variable both within and across national boundaries. Federal legislation can impose some common legal and ethical standards within nations. There is no equivalent body ensuring common standards of health care practice at the transnational level. Furthermore, it is unclear whether international accreditation bodies such as Joint Commission International are setting sufficiently high standards when they evaluate facilities and then provide their 'gold seal of approval'. International accreditation bodies might set baseline standards of practice, but establishing a minimum baseline for provision of health services is very different from demanding and enforcing high standards of professionalism. Preserving continuity of care is a serious challenge when multiple health care providers located in different countries are involved in providing patient care. Legislation related to malpractice, negligence, personal injury and professional standards of care differs across national boundaries and medical tourism companies want legal disputes to be adjudicated in settings where medical tourists face significant barriers to obtaining legal redress after experiencing medically negligent care. Finally, the economic interests of medical tourism companies and destination hospitals generates questions about what information is provided to patients and whether in some circumstances risks are minimised, benefits are exaggerated and profit-seeking is placed before the best interests of patients. *Caveat emptor* is a risky philosophy in most spheres of social interaction but it is particularly dangerous in the realm of health care.

Reports of patients receiving substandard care while abroad and returning home with serious infections and the need for revision surgery and costly follow-up care generate questions about quality of care at some international health care destinations. If increasing numbers of patients travelling abroad for care suffer from postoperative infections, undergo substandard surgery or are otherwise harmed while receiving treatment there might soon be a backlash against medical travel and the promotion of 'bargain-priced' medical care. Recognising possible harms medical travel causes to public health care systems in countries seeking to attract medical tourists, some nations might decide to discard plans to attract large numbers of international patients. Though there are numerous proponents for crossing borders to obtain health care in the global marketplace, there are many reasons to advocate for locally available, affordable, timely, safe, effective and equitable health care. Globalisation affects many dimensions of social and economic life but there is reason to wonder whether globalisation of health services generates as yet not fully understood risks to patients and health systems.

Many patients doubtless arrange safe, competent care abroad. However, a growing body of evidence raises disturbing questions about the quality and safety of medical procedures provided at some international health care destinations. Although destination hospitals, government agencies, medical tourism companies and individual health care providers seeking to market their services promote transnational medical travel, basic questions remain concerning patient safety, quality of care, health equity and effects upon public health systems in destination nations as well as the countries to which patients return after receiving treatment. While a transnational marketplace for health services exists, there is little reason to conclude that the establishment of adequate global ethical frameworks and transnational structures of governance, health law and regulation is accompanying this development.

References

Arellano, A., 2007. Patients Without Borders: The emergence of medical tourism. *International Journal of Health Services*, 37(1), pp. 193–8.

Bennett, B., 2007. Law and Ethics for the Bioeconomy and Beyond. *Journal of Law and Medicine*, 15(1), pp. 7–13.

Bergmark, R., Barr, D. and Garcia, R., 2010. Mexican Immigrants in the US Living Far From the Border May Return to Mexico for Health Services. *Journal of Immigration and Minority Health*, 2(4), pp. 610–14.

Bhatia, V., Arora, P., Parida, A.K., Mittal, A., Pandey, A.K. et al., 2009. Air Travel and Pulmonary Embolism: 'Economy class syndrome'. *The Journal of the Association of Physicians of India*, 57, pp. 412–14.

Birch, D.W., Vu, L., Karmali, S., Stoklossa, C.J. and Sharma, A.M., 2010. Medical Tourism in Bariatric Surgery. *The American Journal of Surgery*, 199(5), pp. 604–8.

Birch, J., Caulfield, R. and Ramakrishnan, V., 2007. The Complications of 'Cosmetic Tourism' – An avoidable burden on the NHS. *Journal of Plastic, Reconstructive & Aesthetic Surgery*, 60(9), pp. 1,075–7.

Budiani-Saberi, D.A. and Delmonico, F.L., 2008. Organ Trafficking and Transplant Tourism: A commentary on the global realities. *American Journal of Transplantation*, 8(5), pp. 925–9.

Burkett, L., 2007. Medical Tourism. Concerns, benefits, and the American legal perspective. *The Journal of Legal Medicine*, 28(2), pp. 223–45.

Chaudhuri, S.K., 2008. Ethics of Medical Tourism. *Journal of the Indian Medical Association*, 106(3), p. 188.

Cheung, I. and Wilson, A., 2007. Arthroplasty Tourism. *Medical Journal of Australia*, 187(11–12), pp. 666–7.

Connell, J., 2006. Medical Tourism: Sea, sun, sand and ... surgery. *Tourism Management*, 27, pp. 1,093–100.

Cortez, N., 2008. Patients Without Borders: The emerging global market for patients and the evolution of modern health care. *Indiana Law Journal*, 83, pp. 71–132.

———, 2009. International Health Care Convergence: The benefits and burdens of market-driven standardization. *Wisconsin International Law Journal*, 26(3), pp. 646–704.

———, 2010. Recalibrating the Legal Risks of Cross-Border Health Care. *Yale Journal of Health Policy, Law, and Ethics*, Winter, pp. 1–87.

Crone, R.K., 2008. Flat Medicine? Exploring trends in the globalization of health care. *Academic Medicine*, 83(2), pp. 117–21.

Delmonico, F.L., 2009. The Hazards of Transplant Tourism. *Clinical Journal of the American Society of Nephrology*, 4(2), pp. 249–50.

Eggertson, L., 2006. Wait-List Weary Canadians Seek Treatment Abroad. *Canadian Medical Association Journal*, 174(9), p. 1,247.

Farrugia, A., 2009. Globalisation and Blood Safety. *Blood Reviews*, 23(3), pp. 123–8.

Feltracco, P., Barbieri, S., Bertamini, F., Michieletto, E. and Ori, C., 2007. Economy Class Syndrome: Still a Recurrent Complication of Long Journeys. *European Journal of Emerging Medicine*, 14(2), pp. 100–103.

Furuya, E.Y., Paez, A., Srinivasan, A., Cooksey, R., Augenbraun, M. et al., 2008. Outbreak of Mycobacterium Abscessus Wound Infections Among 'Lipotourists' from the United States Who Underwent Abdominoplasty in the Dominican Republic. *Clinical Infectious Diseases*, 46(8), pp. 1,181–8.

Garud, A.D., 2005. Medical Tourism and its Impact on our Healthcare. *National Medical Journal of India*, 18(6), pp. 318–19.

Geddes, C.C., Henderson, A., Mackenzie, P., Rodger, S.C., 2008. Outcome of Patients from the West of Scotland Traveling to Pakistan for Living Donor Kidney Transplants. *Transplantation*, 86(8), pp. 1,143–5.

Green, S., 2008. Medical Tourism – A potential growth factor in infection medicine and public health. *Journal of Infection*, 57(5), p. 429.

Handschin, A., Banic, A. and Constantinescu, M., 2007. Pulmonary Embolism after Plastic Surgery Tourism. *Clinical and Applied Thrombosis/Hemostasis*, 13(3), p. 340.

Hanna, S., Saksena, J., Legge, S. and Ware, H., 2009. Sending NHS Patients for Operations Abroad: Is the holiday over? *Annals of the Royal College of Surgeons of England*, 91, pp. 128–30.

Harling, R., Turbitt, D., Millar, M., Ushiro-Lumb, I., Lacey, S. et al., 2007. Passage from India: An outbreak of hepatitis B linked to a patient who acquired infection from health care overseas. *Public Health*, 121(10), pp. 734–41.

Hazarika, I., 2010. Medical Tourism: Its potential impact on the health workforce and health systems in India. *Health Policy Planning*, 25(3), pp. 248–251.

Higgins, R., West, N., Fletcher, S., Stein, A., Lam, F. et al., 2003. Kidney Transplantation in Patients Travelling from the UK to India or Pakistan. *Nephrology Dialysis Transplantation*, 18(4), pp. 851–2.

Inhorn, M.C. and Patrizio, P., 2009. Rethinking Reproductive 'Tourism' as Reproductive 'Exile'. *Fertility and Sterility*, 92(3), pp. 904–6.

Jeevan, R. and Armstrong, A., 2008. Cosmetic Tourism and the Burden on the NHS. *Journal of Plastic, Reconstructive & Aesthetic Surgery*, 61(12), pp. 1,423–4.

Kangas, B., 2002. Therapeutic Itineraries in a Global World: Yemenis and their search for biomedical treatment abroad. *Medical Anthropology*, 21(1), pp. 35–78.

Kiatpongsan, S. and Sipp, D., 2009. Medicine. Monitoring and regulating offshore stem cell clinics. *Science*, 323(5,921), pp. 1,564–5.

Kranhold, K., 1997. US Arrests 19 in Alleged Scheme to Bilk Insurers. *Wall Street Journal*, 15 October, p. 1.

Krishna, B.V., 2010. New Delhi Metallo-Beta-Lactamases: A wake-up call for microbiologists. *Indian Journal of Medical Microbiology*, 28(3), pp. 265–6.

Kumarasamy, K.K., Toleman, M.A., Walsh, T.R., Bagaria, J., Butt, F. et al., 2010. Emergence of a New Antibiotic Resistance Mechanism in India, Pakistan, and the UK: A molecular, biological, and epidemiological study. *Lancet Infectious Diseases*, 10(9), pp. 597–602.

Lee, J.Y., Kearns, R. and Friesen, W., 2010. Seeking Affective Health Care: Korean immigrants' use of homeland medical services. *Health and Place*, 16, pp. 108–15.

Lunt, N. and Carrera, P., 2010. Medical Tourism: Assessing the evidence on treatment abroad. *Maturitas*, 66(1), pp. 27–32.

Lunt, N., Hardey, M. and Mannion, R., 2010. Nip, Tuck and Click: Medical tourism and the emergence of web-based health information. *The Open Medical Informatics Journal*, 4, pp. 1–11.

Mattoo, A. and Rathindran, R., 2006. How Health Insurance Inhibits Trade in Health Care. *Health Affairs*, 25(2), pp. 358–68.

Milstein, A. and Smith, M., 2006. America's New Refugees – Seeking affordable surgery offshore. *New England Journal of Medicine*, 355(16), pp. 1,637–40.

———, 2007. Will the surgical world become flat? *Health Affairs*, 26(1), pp. 137–41.

Mirrer-Singer, P., 2007. Medical Malpractice Overseas: The legal uncertainty surrounding medical tourism. *Law and Contemporary Problems*, 70, pp. 211–32.

Mitka, M., 2009. Surgical Tourism: Some US patients travel abroad for less costly surgery. *Journal of the American Medical Association*, 302(14), p. 1,519.

Moazam, F., Zaman, R.M. and Jafarey, A.M., 2009. Conversations with Kidney Vendors in Pakistan: An ethnographic study. *Hastings Center Report*, 39(3), pp. 29–44.

Muir, A. and Weinbren, M.J., 2010. New Delhi Metallo-Beta-Lactamase: A cautionary tale. *Journal of Hospital Infection*, 75(3), pp. 239–40.

Newman, M., Camberos, A. and Ascherman, J., 2005. Mycobacteria Absessus Outbreak in US Patients Linked to Offshore Surgicenter. *Annals of Plastic Surgery*, 55(1), pp. 107–10.

O'Connor, A., 1997. 21 Arraigned in Cross-Border Fraud Scheme. *Los Angeles Times*, 16 October, p. 23.

Padilla, B.S., 2009. Regulated Compensation for Kidney Donors in the Philippines. *Current Opinion in Organ Transplantation*, 14(2), pp. 120–23.

Radcliffe-Richards, J., Daar, A.S., Guttmann, R.D., Hoffenberg, R., Kennedy, I. et al., 1998. The Case for Allowing Kidney Sales. *The Lancet*, 351(9120), pp. 1,950–52.

Reed, C.M., 2008. Medical Tourism. *Medical Clinics of North America*, 92(6), pp. 1,433–46, xi.

Scheper-Hughes, N., 2000. The Global Traffic in Human Organs. *Current Anthropology*, 41(2), pp. 191–224.

———, 2003. Keeping an Eye on the Global Traffic in Human Organs. *The Lancet*, 361(9,369), pp. 1,645–8.

Sen Gupta, A., 2008. Medical Tourism in India: Winners and losers. *Indian Journal of Medical Ethics*, 5(1), pp. 4–5.

Shroder, S., 2009. Four Accused in Surgery Scheme. *The San Diego Union-Tribune*, 25 April, p. 3.

Svantesson, D.J.B., 2008. From the Airport to the Surgery to the Courtroom – Private international law and medical tourism. *Commonwealth Law Bulletin*, 34(2), pp. 265–76.

Thomas, G. and Krishnan, S., 2010. Effective Public-Private Partnership in Healthcare: Apollo as a cautionary tale. *Indian Journal of Medical Ethics*, 7(1), pp. 2–4.

Turner, L., 2007a. First World Health Care at Third World Prices: Globalization, bioethics and medical tourism. *BioSocieties*, 2, pp. 303–25.

———, 2007b. Medical Tourism: Family medicine and international health-related travel. *Canadian Family Physician*, 53(10), pp. 1,639–41, 46–8.

Wachter, R.M., 2006. The 'Dis-location' of US Medicine – The implications of medical outsourcing. *New England Journal of Medicine*, 354(7), pp. 661–5.

Walker, H. and Brooker, T., 2009. Gelman W. Abdominal Wall Reconstruction Following Removal of a Chronically Infected Mid-Urethral Tape. *International Urogynecology Journal*, 20, pp. 1,273–5.

Whittaker, A., 2008. Pleasure and Pain: Medical travel in Asia. *Global Public Health*, 3(3), pp. 271–90.

Yakupoglu, Y.K., Ozden, E., Dilek, M., Demirbas, A., Adibelli, Z. et al., 2010. Transplantation Tourism: High risk for the recipients. *Clinical Transplantation*, 24(6), pp. 835–8.

Yang, Y., Ani, S., Bartlett, G. and Moazzam, A., 2009. Cosmetic Medical Tourism: Its true cost. *ANZ Journal of Surgery*, 79(s1), p. A60.

Chapter 7

Risks and Challenges for Patients Crossing Borders for Infertility Treatment

Wannes Van Hoof and Guido Pennings

Introduction

Cross-border reproductive care (CBRC) is a distinctive form of medical tourism in which infertile patients cross borders to obtain treatment. Infertility treatments present specific legal, ethical, practical, psychological and even medical issues that warrant reflection beyond the scope of general medical tourism. Hence, there are specific risks and challenges for patients who cross borders for infertility treatment.

There is a general lack of empirical data on the prevalence of CBRC (Inhorn and Gürtin, 2011). In the most elaborate study to date data from 46 clinics in six countries (Belgium, Czech Republic, Denmark, Slovenia, Spain and Switzerland) was gathered about 1,230 cross-border patients from 49 countries. During one calendar month between October 2008 and March 2009 these clinics conducted a survey on every foreign patients they treated (Shenfield et al., 2010). Based on this study, the European Society for Human Reproduction and Embryology (ESHRE) estimated that at least 12,000–15,000 patients cross borders for fertility treatment within Europe each year and that this number will continue to rise. No reliable data is available for North America, but physicians estimate it to be a widespread phenomenon (Hughes and DeJean, 2010). Several countries in Asia, most notably India, are often named as popular destination countries for controversial treatments like commercial surrogacy (Humbyrd, 2009). More recently, South American private clinics have discovered the market for fertility care (Smith et al., 2010).

The same conditions that enable patients to travel for medical treatments also facilitate fertility tourism: access to information (internet), cheap flights, hospital networks, patient's rights and attitude change, portability of health insurance, marketing by clinics, commercialisation of medical services and so on. However, the nature of infertility treatment makes it unlikely that, even when there are few limitations on travelling, infertile patients would prefer to travel. Infertility treatment is a physical and emotional burden: an unfulfilled child wish, repeated disappointments and failures, uncertainty, strain on a relationship etcetera (Boivin et al., 2012). Given that patients appreciate coordination, accessibility and continuity of care, it follows that they want to continue treatment locally as long as possible (Dancet et al., 2011).

The reasons why some infertile patients do travel can be summed up as legal or access difficulties at home (Pennings et al., 2008). Legal difficulties occur when certain treatments (like egg donation or surrogacy) are forbidden in a country or when specific groups (such as single persons or homosexual couples) are denied treatment. Access difficulties occur when waiting lists are too long, out-of-pocket costs are too high, expertise or equipment is lacking, good quality care is unavailable or when people have specific desires (for example, to have an anonymous or identifiable gamete donor). The reasons why patients travel largely depend on the legal situation and the quality of care in the home country. The ESHRE study found that 80.2 per cent of German patients, 70. 6 per cent of Italian patients and 64.5 per cent of French patients travelled for legal reasons whereas 53.0 per cent of Dutch patients travelled for better quality of care and 34.0 per cent of UK patients experienced access difficulties at home (Shenfield et al., 2010). The desire for timely and affordable treatment with donor gametes is the most important motivation to travel for UK patients (Culley et al., 2011).

In this chapter, we will address the main risks and challenges for cross-border patients. While this means that we will focus on the (potential) negative aspects of CBRC, we do not consider CBRC as a negative phenomenon in itself. CBRC increases reproductive autonomy. Reproductive autonomy refers to the right of people to decide when, how, with whom and how many children they will have. When infertility treatment is not available at home or when a treatment is forbidden by the law of their home country, it increases the patients' autonomy when they can obtain treatment abroad. The ESHRE Task Force on Ethics and Law argued that the principle of reproductive autonomy justifies transgression of the general obligation to obey the law of one's country in a number of situations as long as safety, efficacy and welfare of the patient and the future child is taken into consideration (Pennings et al., 2008).

Main risks and challenges in CBRC

CBRC has a bad name. Many organisations warn their members about travelling to another country. Also governmental organisations such as the Human Fertilisation and Embryology Authority in the United Kingdom find it necessary to inform their citizens about the risks involved. We analysed the statements of 5 major organisations – that is, European Society of Human Reproduction and Embryology (ESHRE); Human Fertilisation and Embryology Authority (HFEA); Donor Conception Network; International Federation of Gynecology and Obstetrics (FIGO); and Infertility Consumer Support for Infertility (iCSi) – on the types of risks and challenges and composed the following list:

- Violation of, or non-compliance with, safety standards (multiple pregnancy, donor screening, ovarian hyperstimulation syndrome (OHSS));
- Violation of, or non-compliance with, quality standards (success rates);

- Confidentiality of patient information (patient medical records);
- Lack or insufficiency of psychosocial and medical counselling (language and culture);
- Financial implications (real cost, reimbursement and so on);
- Differences in gamete donation arrangements and surrogacy (anonymity, legal rights and obligations);
- Legal recourse after treatment (malpractice, indemnification, insurance and so on).

Several strategies have been developed to deal with these issues. The EU has enacted laws and directives to guarantee safety of care and to protect patient rights. ESHRE published a good practice guide for CBRC specifically directed at clinics and practitioners (Shenfield et al., 2011). Outside of the EU, the American Bar Association has issued good policy guidelines to deal with the legal diversity concerning commercial surrogacy in the USA (Kindregan and Snyder, 2008). Health insurers worldwide are offering portable insurance packages that provide financial and legal support for cross-border patients.

Like all statements in scientific research, the assumed dangers of CBRC should be corroborated by empirical evidence. At the moment, a lot of anecdotal evidence circulates on the internet as well as in academic literature and, given the possible conflict of interest of the sources of the rumours, these should be handled with care. There are, for instance, few reports of cross-border women being overstimulated or gamete donors being improperly screened in countries with many cross-border patients. There have been reports of anecdotal overstimulation of egg donors in clinics in some countries (for example, Romania and Ukraine), where women are paid per egg rather than compensated for their time and inconvenience (Barnett and Smith, 2006). However, before one starts frightening patients with all kinds of horror stories, it would be wise to collect the necessary evidence to support the allegations.

Safety: Multiple Pregnancies

The most serious harm associated with CBRC is the risk of multiple pregnancies. Multiple pregnancy leads to a strong increase in obstetric complications, perinatal morbidity, maternal and child mortality rate, congenital malformations, pre-term birth, long-term social, psychological and financial difficulties. In a way, the occurrence of this side effect of ART is a test case for the moral quality of the field (Pennings, 2000). The most recent report of pregnancy rates in Europe indicates that there are still huge differences: in 2008, twin pregnancies after IVF or ICSI occurred in 7 per cent of cases in Sweden, 11.5 per cent of cases in Belgium, 23.8 per cent of cases in Spain and 24.5 per cent of cases in the UK (Ferraretti et al., 2012).

It is often claimed that CBRC is responsible for a higher rate of multiple pregnancies. This accusation may be partially caused by the fact that some clinics, mainly outside of Europe, explicitly refer to the fact that they do not have to abide by the same guidelines regarding the number of embryos to transfer (Mulay and Gibson, 2006). The allegation seems to be confirmed by other data. Pennings et al. (2009) provided some evidence for a higher number of embryos transferred in cross-border patients. However, one should take into account that the number of embryos transferred depends on the number of previous unsuccessful cycles and on the age of the patient. On both criteria, cross-border patients as a group differ from the local population. Many cross-border patients have had previous treatments and present difficult cases. In general, infertility patients are looking for the procedure that is most likely to result in a pregnancy and they do not see multiple pregnancy as an unfavourable outcome (Newton et al., 2007). One may expect that cross-border patients, given the price they have to pay for their treatment (in Belgium, one IVF cycle including tests and drugs costs around €5,000 for non-reimbursed patients) and the fact that it is a last chance intervention in many cases, will insist even more than ordinary patients on multiple embryo transfer. However, on this specific point, it is important that good practice guidelines are followed.

The study by McKelvey et al. (2009) is often cited to prove that CBRC causes high order multiple pregnancies which results in additional costs for national health care systems. They stated that a quarter of the high order pregnancies in their clinic were caused by multiple embryo transfers abroad. However, they showed merely that patients returning to the UK had fewer embryo reductions in case of higher order multiple pregnancies (33 per cent of cross-border patients versus 51.4 per cent of local patients). They did not show that these patients also had more embryos transferred than in the UK. In fact, the multiple pregnancy rate is very high in the UK compared to other European countries (Ferraretti et al., 2012). Whereas CBRC is often cited as leading to more multiple pregnancies, one might also argue that patients from countries with a high multiple pregnancy rate should, for their own safety, seek treatment in countries with a low multiple pregnancy rate. Whether or not CBRC jeopardises patient's health depends on the starting conditions at home.

Prevention of multiple pregnancy is part of good clinical practice and protection of the patient. On a national level, multiple pregnancy has successfully been managed by linking reimbursement to a SET (single embryo transfer) policy in Sweden, Belgium and other countries. International accreditation should also be linked to an SET policy in clinics.

Safety: Complications

The principle of non-maleficence dictates that all patients should receive safe and effective treatment wherever they go. The harms associated with CBRC are mostly multiple pregnancy and to a lesser extent OHSS. OHSS occurs mostly in mild forms, in which case it is relatively harmless, but in about 1 per cent of hormonally stimulated women severe OHSS occurs, which carries a very small risk of a life-threatening complication (Delvigne, 2009). However, this danger may be referred to the past if research confirms that new stimulation protocols can reduce the risk of OHSS to almost zero (Mertes and Pennings, 2011).

Every patient who needs stimulation is to be considered potentially at risk for OHSS (Delvigne, 2009). In the case of CBRC, the monitoring of OHSS is complicated because its symptoms appear sometime after the treatment. Cross-border patients should be instructed on what to do in case of abnormal fever, pelvic pain, vaginal bleeding or more severe symptoms of OHSS (De Sutter, 2011). When severe OHSS occurs, patients may need to be helped by a local clinic to prevent further harm and complications. One physician with extensive experience in treating foreign patients wrote:

> Although collaboration with foreign 'home' clinics is excellent in 99% of cases, once a patient with severe OHSS travelled 200 km back to the centre because their local hospital refused to help them, telling them that if they went abroad for their treatment, they were on their own and should also take full responsibility if something goes wrong. This situation is both unfortunate and potentially dangerous for the patient's health. Although this case is exceptional, the centre always instructs patients to look for 'sympathetic' local clinics before they start treatment. (De Sutter 2011, p. 655)

From an ethical point of view, this home clinic demonstrated a highly dubious attitude. Doctors have a duty to help persons in need even if those persons are (partially) responsible for their own condition. Mancini et al. (2011) reported a case of an Italian woman whose ectopic pregnancy after egg donor treatment in Spain (which is illegal under Italian law) was only diagnosed just in time because the woman had trouble finding a local physician willing to help. Additionally, she did not disclose that she engaged in CBRC for law evasion when she contacted a local physician. It was only when the foreign clinic contacted the local physician that the proper diagnose could be made. It is important that local doctors take an open stance regarding treatment abroad (even when they disapprove) because only then patients will contact and inform them about what they have done.

Safety: Collaboration Between Providers

Good cooperation with a physician at home ensures sufficient follow-up care and continuity of care. Cooperation may include exchange of information and shared treatment. Information exchange is a two-way street: information from the referring centres to the receiving centres can prevent unnecessary testing and inappropriate treatments. Information from the treating centres abroad to the local doctor may improve the follow-up of the patients when complications occur or pregnancy is achieved. For this to be possible, patients should be provided with adequate information about their prior treatment (FIGO, 2010). In order to facilitate such information sharing between health care providers, all kinds of devices or instruments are designed such as an internationally accessible electronic patient file. However, these solutions always hold risks for privacy and data confidentiality and fail-safe solutions still have to be found.

When patients have their infertility treatment abroad, they are to a certain degree socially isolated and have less psychological support from friends and family. Understandably, some patients want to shorten the stay abroad by doing part of the treatment at home. Data from the ESHRE study indicate that not all patients did receive help from their local doctor (Table 7.1). It is note-worthy that Italian and German patients, whose main reason to travel was to evade the restrictive legislation of their home country, are helped more often than Dutch patients, who travel for better quality care. Collaboration between providers mostly seems to be a question of goodwill. For Dutch physicians, it has been suggested that they do not like to be 'errand boys' for their foreign colleagues (Van Hoof and Pennings, 2013). When a restrictive law is in place, the personal opinion of the local physicians on the morality of the law may determine their willingness to collaborate.

Dividing treatment between different clinics also creates new risks and challenges with regard to communication between clinics and adjustment of procedures. Although the available evidence does not indicate major problems in this regard, the discrepancies between what some doctors provide and what other doctors expect in terms of information suggest that there is more work to be done (Hughes and DeJean, 2010).

Table 7.1   Help received from local doctor (per cent)

Country	No help	Drug prescription	Cycle monitoring	Both
France	21.0	37.0	6.0	36.0
Germany	18.3	9.1	31.7	40.9
Italy	44.7	20.5	10.7	24.2
Netherlands	65.0	19.6	4.2	11.2
Norway	27.1	5.1	37.3	30.5
United Kingdom	54.7	15.1	15.1	15.1

Source: Unpublished data from the 2010 ESHRE Taskforce study on CBRC.

Safety: Reliable Information

When patients run out of options at home, they have to select a clinic abroad. The two most important sources of information to select a clinic are the internet (41 per cent) and the local doctor (41 per cent) (Shenfield et al., 2010). Individuals contemplating CBRC who rely on the internet for information find it hard to obtain accessible, accurate and reliable information (Blyth, 2010). Patients run the risk of choosing the wrong clinic because there is no reliable information available. Many clinics, for example, offer confusing and exaggerated information on success rates (Spar, 2006). For infertility treatment, success rates largely depend on patient characteristics such as age and indication, and they vary considerably across different treatments. Clinics can easily manipulate data to appear more successful. For the patients, this results in a lack of transparency. However, unreliable website information is not a problem specific for cross-border patients. All patients, regardless of whether they look for a clinic outside their own country, are confronted with this problem.

Patients' organisations should empower patients by providing them with reliable information. However, it is challenging, if not impossible, for any individual or professional organisation to always have reliable current knowledge and information about the entire range of treatment possibilities abroad (Thorn and Dill, 2010). A more comprehensive solution would be to ensure access to 'official' data that allows patients to compare clinics. The Fertility Clinic Success Rate and Certification Act of 1992 in the United States mandates that clinics performing ART annually provide data for all procedures to the Centers for Disease Control and Prevention (CDC). These reports are explicitly meant to help patients to find and choose a clinic. It would improve the present situation considerably when clinics would be obliged by law to put a link to the CDC website on their own website. At present, many clinics advertise with all kinds of statements (such as 'better than the national average') but patients do not know how they can verify these statements (Hawkins, 2013). A comparable system exists in the United Kingdom where the Human Fertilisation and Embryology Authority website explains how success rates should be interpreted and also provides a tool on how to choose a clinic. Similar structures in other countries would largely eliminate this issue from the list of potential challenges for all patients, including cross-border patients.

When patients reach a stage where further treatment is no longer available at home (because it is illegal, technologically too advanced and so on), their local physician can help by referring them to a good clinic abroad. A fairly large number of doctors (41 per cent of patients indicate their doctor as a source of information) provide this support to their patients (Shenfield et al., 2010). In a Canadian survey, 52 per cent of doctors always recommend a destination country but only 21 per cent recommend a specific provider (Hughes and DeJean, 2010). However, direct referral assumes that the local physician is aware of the situation in another country and is familiar with at least one clinic there. This is not always the case. One may even question the appropriateness of a direct referral. Two situations should be mentioned. More and more clinics become part of hospital chains with branches abroad. Referral will then evidently be to the affiliated clinics. This is not necessarily a bad thing (assuming that this clinic works according to the same standard of good clinical practice) but it may restrain the patient's freedom of choice. Moreover, this clinic may be suboptimal (more expensive, less successful and so on) compared to other clinics in that country. Still, an unguided choice may be worse. Secondly, there is anecdotal evidence about fee-splitting; that is, the referring doctor receives a fee solely for referring the patient to a specific colleague. This practice, which is condemned as unethical, undoes the benefits of direct referral because it generates a conflict of interest in the doctor that may run counter to the best interest of the patient (Pennings et al., 2008). Besides the problems mentioned above, direct referral may also be either against the law in some countries (like Germany) or against the conscience of the doctor. By referring the patient, and thus helping her to evade the law, the physician may consider him/herself as an accessory of some kind. The Human Genetics Commission in the United Kingdom recommended in 2006 that the HFEA should explore ways to prevent clinics from preparing or otherwise colluding with individuals seeking treatments abroad that are prohibited within the UK (Human Genetics Commission, 2006). Also the ESHRE Task Force on Cross Border Reproductive Care stated that when a home practitioner refers a patient to a specific clinic, he or she shares a responsibility for the general standards used in that clinic (Shenfield et al., 2011). A possible solution to this problem is that professional and patients organisations actively collect and provide information on foreign clinics.

Within the discussion on information, one tends to overlook the possible burden of making arrangements for international travelling. This indirectly leads to a selection of higher educated people who find their way on the internet and speak at least one foreign language. In the field of medical tourism, this problem is solved by host clinics offering package deals to patients including visa, plane tickets, translators, transport from the airport and so on. This seems to be less common in infertility treatment but it surely facilitates things for the patient.

Counselling

Information provision and counselling are important to promote informed consent and thus patient autonomy. Good counselling ensures that all parties are fully informed, aware of the long term consequences of their treatment and prepared for (supported through) the mental strains of infertility treatment. Especially when donor gametes or surrogacy services are used, counselling about long-term social and psychological consequences is indispensable (Thorn et al., 2012). Given the fact that we are talking about highly personal and sensitive topics, this might become very difficult when the counselling has to be done in a language that is not the patient's mother tongue and in a cultural setting that may deviate strongly from the patient's own background. Moreover, a foreign counsellor or physician will have a hard time to fully inform patients due to a lack of knowledge about the patients' personal and medical history, social and cultural differences and so on. There is little data on counselling and CBRC, but the data that has been published so far is mostly reassuring (Hudson et al., 2011; Pennings et al., 2009; Shenfield et al., 2010). Most European patients were able to receive information in their own language when they were treated abroad (Table 7.2). Given the enormous diversity of patients and languages, it is unrealistic to expect clinics to have a translator for every possible patient. Nevertheless, patients should receive basic counselling in a language they understand reasonably well. If this is impossible, one should refuse treatment.

Table 7.2   **Information received in own language (per cent)**

Country	No	Unsatisfactory prescription	Satisfactory
Belgium	6.6	0.9	92.5
Czech Republic	2.5	1.2	96.3
Denmark	27.2	0.0	72.8
Slovenia	1.6	12.7	85.7
Spain	5.3	1.0	93.7

Source: Unpublished data from the 2010 ESHRE Taskforce study on CBRCAt the same time, we also know very little about uptake and quality of counselling in normal settings. There are significant differences in counselling practices among countries (who does it? What is the goal? To whom is it offered?) (Blyth, 2012). Moreover, many countries have large minority groups inside their borders that have a different cultural, religious and language background that may render local counselling also very difficult. In addition, many clinics with a considerable population of foreign patients have attracted doctors from countries representing the main countries of origin. It seems again to show prejudice when the point about the difficulty of counselling is advanced specifically against CBRC.

Table 7.2 shows that the overwhelming majority of foreign patients were satisfied with the counselling they received. However, one should take into account that not all patients take up the offer or want to have counselling. Counselling is a broad term. When it is interpreted as information provision, there are minimum standards with regard to informed consent: a responsibility shared by local and foreign caretakers (Thorn et al., 2012). When it is interpreted as psychosocial counselling, it should be available with a minimal threshold and with regard for the specific profile of a cross-border patient (Blyth et al., 2011).

Legal Conflicts

Many patients engage in CBRC to evade a restrictive law of their home country. When these patients return home, they may face practical problems because of the legal diversity (Van Hoof and Pennings, 2012). For example, when gamete donation is prohibited or same sex couples are denied access to assisted reproduction, the partner who is not genetically related to the child will not have parental rights in his/her home country.

When patients from countries with identifiable gamete donation systems travel to countries where anonymous donation is the standard, their future children (if they are informed about their donor conception) will grow up in a society where knowledge of genetic origins is deemed important and where locally conceived donor children do have access to this information. Obviously, patients will have to balance this disadvantage against faster treatment. At the same time, other patients will move to other countries precisely to have either identifiable or anonymous donation that is not available at home.

Other legal conflicts confront patients with more serious problems. In the case of international commercial surrogacy, there are numerous reports of children who are 'stuck' abroad because the surrogacy contract the commissioning couple engaged in abroad is not recognised at home. In that case, the birth mother (the surrogate) is considered to be the legal mother by the home country while the reverse position is adopted in the country of destination (Van Hoof and Pennings, 2012). This has happened to commissioning couples from Belgium, Germany, Ireland, France, Japan the UK and elsewhere. All commissioning couples from countries where commercial surrogacy is not regulated or banned entirely face similar problems after international commercial surrogacy. In the United Kingdom, there is a well-documented case of a couple who went to Ukraine in 2008. They used the husband's sperm to fertilise a donor egg and the Ukrainian surrogate mother gave birth to twins. UK laws allow altruistic surrogacy but condemns commercialisation and bans commercial brokering and advertising (Gamble, 2009). The commissioning couple signed a commercial surrogacy contract in the Ukraine, which included payment of £23,000 and gave them parental rights under Ukrainian law. However, under UK law the mother who gives birth is recognised as the legal mother and her husband as the legal father. The effect of the conflict between Ukrainian and UK laws was that the parental status of both couples was abdicated. The only way to recognise the children in the UK was with a parental order, which is used to assign parenthood to commissioning couples in altruistic surrogacy. This was the main point of discussion in the UK courts: the commercial nature of the surrogacy was in direct conflict with the law. The judge ultimately decided to grant the parental order to ensure the welfare of the child (Theis et al., 2009).

Recognition of a child born through commercial surrogacy abroad can be difficult even when it is regulated at home. Most countries recognise two ways to gain citizenship: being born (or spending a certain amount of time) in the country (*ius soli*) or being the genetic offspring of a citizen (*ius sanguini*). In the case of international commercial surrogacy, it is possible that the child is neither born on the territory nor genetically related to a citizen. The US Department of State issued a statement in which they warned US citizens that 'even if local law recognises a surrogacy agreement and finds that U.S. parents are the legal parents of a child conceived through ART, if the U.S. citizen parents do not have a biological connection to the child, the child will not be a U.S. citizen at birth' (US Department of State, 2012). Their advice to patients having ART treatment abroad is to consult with an immigration attorney first. Even more remarkable, and quite worrying, is the fact that the Department of State says that it is aware 'of cases of foreign fertility clinics that have substituted alternate donor sperm and eggs when the U.S. parents' genetic material turned out not to be viable' (US Department of State, 2012). If we read this correctly, the gametes of the would-be parents were switched with other gametes when conception failed; and this without telling the parents. Currently, the long and difficult road of adoption remains the only option to deal with these problems.

Reimbursement and Costs

The principle of justice dictates that there should be equitable access to basic health care without excessive burden. The extent to which the principle of justice applies to infertility treatment depends on the status of infertility treatment: is it part of basic health care or not? Since the right to procreate is a human right, it seems evident to classify infertility treatment as basic health care. However, there are several arguments to the contrary: infertility does not lead to physical harm, treatment often does not cure infertility, there are limited resources to be distributed in any health care system and infertility treatment is expensive, there are other parties involved in infertility treatments (future child, medical personnel, gamete donors, surrogates) whose rights may supersede a person's right to procreate and so on. In a nuanced form the principle of justice dictates that those infertility treatments that are considered to be morally sound and reasonable should be available and affordable for everyone. Financial means should not be a criterion.

The relevant question here is how CBRC affects the principle of justice with regard to infertility treatment. One should distinguish between people who travel because of law evasion and people who travel because the cost of treatment in their home country is too high (Hudson et al., 2011). The colloquial criticism of CBRC is that 'only rich people can go abroad'. It is obviously correct that one requires money to obtain treatment abroad but that is also true when no reimbursement is offered at home. Poor people in countries without a reimbursement system may be better off when they travel to another country, even when they have to pay the full price and have to cover the extra costs of travel and stay. The price differences of IVF are considerable, even within Europe (Connolly et al., 2010). So, contrary to the criticism, CBRC increases access for patients from countries without reimbursement through health insurance. Moreover, one should avoid a 'morality of envy': 'if I cannot have it, no one should'. It implies a form of blaming the victim, since patients who cannot access treatment at home first are then denied the option of going abroad as well. Patients who make use of CBRC for law evasion already feel abandoned by their country and the process of CBRC is very difficult for them due to a lack of support (Zanini, 2011).

There is an easy solution that ensures that CBRC increases justice for treatments that are considered legal in the home country: health insurers should reimburse the costs of treatment abroad. Reproductive autonomy and justice are increased through portability of health insurance. The European Union is taking steps in this direction with the recent directive on the application of patients' rights in cross-border health care (2011/24/EU). This directive gives patients the right to be reimbursed without prior authorisation for care in any EU Member State up to the limit to which the patient is entitled according to the legislation of home country. This directive means that patients who live in a country with permissive policies, like the UK and the Netherlands, will be reimbursed abroad as well, but patients from countries with restrictive policies like Italy, Germany and France still have to pay themselves. The directive ensures that when infertility treatment is judged to be a part of basic health care, it is reimbursed across borders. However, the decision whether or not the principle of justice applies to infertility treatment is left to the individual state. From the ESHRE study, we learn that before the implementation of the directive, only patients from the Netherlands received partial (44 per cent) or full (17 per cent) reimbursement of their treatment cost (Shenfield et al., 2010). On a practical level, arranging reimbursement may prove to be an administrative burden for patients. A recent review of Dutch internet forums on infertility treatment in Belgium indicated that patients help each other play the system to ensure maximal reimbursement (Van Hoof and Pennings, 2013).

A final challenge for cross-border patients is to obtain a relatively accurate estimation of the costs. This is difficult for two reasons. Firstly, it turns out that many clinics do not mention their prices on their websites (Hawkins, 2013). Secondly, price comparisons between different clinics are very hard to make since clinics frequently bundle treatment into packages differently. Moreover, it is not always clear whether everything is included or whether parts like counselling or medication should be paid for separately. Again, standardisation in presentation would be helpful.

Conclusion

Patients who cross borders for infertility treatment face many risks and challenges, but if all parties involved (patients, physicians, clinics and policy makers) adhere to the general ethical principles (reproductive autonomy, non-maleficence and justice), there are solutions to most problems associated with CBRC. Many risks and challenges can be prevented when patient groups, professional societies and governmental institutes educate patients about what information to seek and how to evaluate this information. All risks and challenges associated with CBRC can be prevented by adopting less restrictive laws and providing good quality infertility care at home.

Many predicted risks did not materialise. It is obviously important that further research is done on the actual experiences of cross-border patients but one should be wary about gratuitous accusations. Many doctors seem to believe that only they offer adequate care. It seems that, at least within Europe, no major problems arise with cross-border infertility treatment. Since cross-border treatment increases justice (in case of restrictive legislation and expensive treatment in one's home country) and autonomy for the patients, it seems that the right way forward is not to emphasise the dangers of going abroad but to adopt measures to empower patients in order to reduce possible dangers.

References

Barnett, A. and Smith, H., 2006. Cruel Cost of the Human Egg Trade. *The Observer*, 30 April.

Blyth, E., 2010. Fertility Patients' Experiences of Cross-Border Reproductive Care. *Fertility and Sterility*, 94(1), pp. e11–15.

———, 2012. Guidelines for Infertility Counselling in Different Countries: Is there an emerging trend? *Human Reproduction*, 27(7), pp. 2,046–57.

Blyth, E., Thorn, P. and Wischmann, T., 2011. CBRC and Psychosocial Counselling: Assessing needs and developing an ethical framework for practice. *Reproductive BioMedicine Online*, 23(5), pp. 642–51.

Boivin, J., Domar, A.D., Shapiro, D.B., Wischmann, T.H., Fauser, B. et al., 2012. Tackling Burden in ART: An integrated approach for medical staff. *Human Reproduction*, 27(4), pp. 941–50.

Connolly, M.P., Hoorens, S. and Chambers, G.M., 2010. The Costs and Consequences of Assisted Reproductive Technology: An economic perspective. *Human Reproduction Update*, 16(6), pp. 603–13.

Culley, L., Hudson, N., Rapport, F., Blyth, E., Norton, W. et al., 2011. Crossing Borders for Fertility Treatment: Motivations, destinations and outcomes of UK fertility travellers. *Human Reproduction*, 26(9), pp. 2,373–81.

Dancet, E.A.F., van Empel, I.W.H., Rober, P., Nelen, W.L.D.M., Kremer, J.A.M. et al., 2011. Patient-Centred Infertility Care: A qualitative study to listen to the patients' voice. *Human Reproduction*, 26, pp. 827–33.

De Sutter, P., 2011. Considerations for Clinics and Practitioners Treating Foreign Patients with Assisted Reproductive Technology: Lessons from experiences at Ghent University Hospital, Belgium. *Reproductive BioMedicine Online*, 23, pp. 652–6.

Delvigne, A., 2009. Epidemiology of OHSS. *Reproductive Biomedicine Online*, 19(1), pp. 8–13.

Donor Conception Network, 2010. *Donor Conception Treatment Outside the UK*. Updated January 2010.

Ferraretti, A.P., Goossens, V., de Mouzon, J., Bhattacharya, S., Castilla, J.A. et al., 2012. Assisted Reproductive Technology in Europe 2008 – Results generated from European registers from ESHRE. *Human Reproduction*, 27(9), pp. 2,571–84.

Gamble, N., 2009. Crossing the Line: The legal and ethical problems of foreign surrogacy. *Reproductive Biomedicine Online*, 19(2), pp. 151–2.

Hawkins, J.S., 2013. Selling ART: An empirical assessment of advertising on fertility clinics' websites. *Indiana Law Journal*, 88, pp. 1147–1179.

Hudson, N., Culley, L., Blyth, E., Norton, W., Rapport, F. et al., 2011. Cross-Border Reproductive Care: A review of the literature. *Reproductive BioMedicine Online*, 22, pp. 673–85.

Hughes, E.J. and DeJean, D., 2010. Cross-Border Fertility Services in North America: A survey of Canadian and American providers. *Fertility and Sterility*, 94(1), pp. e16–e19.

Human Fertilisation and Embryology Authority, 2009. *Considering Treatment Abroad: Issues and risks.* [online] Available at: <http://www.hfea.gov.uk/95.html> [Accessed 23 December 2103].

Human Genetics Commission, 2006. *Making Babies: Reproductive decisions and genetic technologies.* London: Human Genetics Commission.

Humbyrd, C., 2009. Fair Trade International Surrogacy. *Developing World Bioethics*, 9(3), pp. 111–18.

Inhorn, M.C. and Gürtin, Z.B., 2011. Cross-Border Reproductive Care: A future research agenda. *Reproductive Biomedicine Online*, 23(5), pp. 665–76.

International Consumer Support for Infertility, 2008. *Travelling Abroad for Assisted Reproductive Technology (ART) Treatment.*

International Federation of Gynecology and Obstetrics (FIGO), 2010. Cross-Border Reproductive Services. *International Journal of Gynecology and Obstetrics*, 111(2), pp. 190–91.

Kindregan, C.P. and Snyder, S.H., 2008. Clarifying the Law of ART: The new American Bar Association Model Act governing assisted reproductive technology. *Family Law Quarterly*, 42(2), pp. 203–29.

Mancini, F., Clua, E., Martínez, F., Battaglia, C., Veiga, A. et al., 2011. Heterotopic Pregnancy in a Cross Border Oocyte Donation Patient: The importance of cooperation between centers. *Fertility and Sterility*, 95(7), pp. e13–15.

McKelvey, A., David A.L., Shenfield, F. and Jauniaux, E.R., 2009. The Impact of Cross-Border Reproductive Care or 'Fertility Tourism' on NHS Maternity Services. *British Journal of Obstetrics and Gynaecology*, 116(11), pp. 1,520–23.

Mertes, H. and Pennings, G., 2011. Ethical Concerns Eliminated: Safer stimulation protocols and egg banking. *American Journal of Bioethics*, 11(9), pp. 33–5.

Mulay, S. and Gibson, E., 2006. Marketing of Assisted Human Reproduction and the Indian State. *Development*, 49(4), pp. 84–93.

Newton, C.R., McBride, J., Feyles, V., Tekpetey, F. and Power, S., 2007. Factors Affecting Patients' Attitudes Toward Single- and Multiple-Embryo Transfer. *Fertility and Sterility*, 87(2), pp. 269–78.

Pennings, G., 2000. Multiple Pregnancies: A test case for the moral quality of medically assisted reproduction. *Human Reproduction*, 15(12), pp. 2,466–9.

———, 2011. Evaluating the Welfare of the Child in Same-Sex Families. *Human Reproduction*, 26(7), pp. 1,609–15.

Pennings, G., Autin, C., Decleer, W., Delbaere, A., Delbeke, L. et al., 2009. Cross-Border Reproductive Care in Belgium. *Human Reproduction*, 24(12), pp. 3,108–18.

Pennings, G., de Wert, G., Shenfield, F., Cohen, J., Tarlatzis, B. et al., 2008. ESHRE Task Force on Ethics and Law 15: Cross-border reproductive care. *Human Reproduction*, 23(10), pp. 2,182–4.

Shenfield, F., de Mouzon, J., Pennings, G., Ferraretti, A.P., Nyboe Andersen, A. et al., 2010. Cross Border Reproductive Care in Six European Countries. *Human Reproduction*, 25(6), pp. 1,361–8.

Shenfield, F., Pennings, G., De Mouzon, J., Ferraretti, A.P. and Goossens, V., 2011. ESHRE's Good Practice Guide for Cross-Border Reproductive Care for Centers and Practitioners. *Human Reproduction*, 26(7), pp. 1,625–7.

Smith, E., Behrmann, J., Martin, C. and Williams-Jones, B., 2010. Reproductive Tourism in Argentina: Clinic accreditation and its implications for consumers, health professionals and policy makers. *Developing World Bioethics*, 10(2), pp. 59–69.

Spar, D., 2006. *The Baby Business: How Money, Science, and Politics Drive the Commerce of Conception*. Boston, Massachusetts: Harvard Business Press.

Theis, L., Gamble, N. and Ghevaert, L., 2009. Re X and Y: 'A trek through a thorn forest'. *Family Law*, 39(March), pp. 239–43.

Thorn, P. and Dill, S., 2010. The Role of Patients' Organizations in Cross-Border Reproductive Care. *Fertility and Sterility*, 94(1), pp. e23–4.

Thorn, P., Wischmann, T. and Blyth, E., 2012. Cross-Border Reproductive Services – Suggestions for ethically based minimum standards of care in Europe. *Journal of Psychosomatic Obstetrics and Gynecology*, 33(1), pp. 1–6.

US Department of State., 2012. *Important Information for U.S. Citizens Considering the Use of Assisted Reproductive Technology (ART) Abroad*. [online] Available at: <http://travel.state.gov/law/citizenship/citizenship_5177.html> [Accessed 23 December 2013].

Van Hoof, W. and Pennings, G., 2012. Extraterritorial Laws for Cross-Border Reproductive Care: The issue of legal diversity. *European Journal of Health Law*, 19(2), pp. 187–200.

———, 2013. Reflections of Dutch Patients on IVF Treatment in Belgium: A qualitative analysis of internet forums. *Human Reproduction*, 28(4), pp. 1,013–22.

Zanini, G., 2011. Abandoned by the State, Betrayed by the Church: Italian experiences of cross-border reproductive care. *Reproductive BioMedicine Online*, 23(5), pp. 565–72.

PART III
Migrating Medical Expertise

Chapter 8

'Real Nursing Work' versus 'Charting and Sweet Talking': The Challenges of Incorporation into US Urban Health Care Settings for Indian Immigrant Nurses

Sheba George

Introduction

The global migration of labour is profoundly shaped by two trends: the first being, migration from economically less wealthy nations to the richer nations and the second being a gendered specificity, in that more women than men tend to migrate (Toro-Morn and Alicea, 2004). The increasing immigration of health care workers to the United States reflects both of these trends, particularly in the field of nursing (Aiken et al., 2004; Xu, 2006). A shortage of nurses in the USA in the 1960s resulted in heavy recruitment of nurses from Asian countries, especially after the passing of the Immigration and Nationality Act of 1965. The trend still persists and is increasing: 6 per cent of new US nurses in 2000 were immigrants whereas 15 per cent were immigrants in 2004 (Redfoot and Houser, 2005). Although immigrant nurses compose only a small but increasing percentage of the nursing work force in the United States, they are a critical source of labour for urban hospitals, particularly safety net hospitals with a largely underserved, multiracial patient base (Arends-Kunning, 2006).

Indian nurses, in particular, have been recruited to meet such a labour demand. However, there is very little information on the experiences of these immigrant nurses – a mostly female, racial/ethnic[1] minority labour force. The objective of this chapter is to examine the work experiences of Indian immigrant nurses in the United States and the challenges they face in becoming incorporated into their new work settings, particularly in urban areas.

---

1 All names of participants are pseudonyms.

Background and Significance

Immigrant Health Care Providers and Health Disparities

A key theme in many recent health policy discussions in the US has been on the relationship between quality of care and health disparities. Upon the request of the United States Congress, the Institute of Medicine (IOM), part of the non-partisan Academy of Sciences, conducted a review of the literature on racial and ethnic health disparities and published their findings in the report entitled 'Unequal Treatment: Confronting Racial and Ethnic Disparities in Health Care' (Smedley, Stith and Nelson, 2003). This study found that racial and ethnic minorities in the US are less likely to receive needed medical care and experience a lower quality of care, even when insurance status, income, age and severity of conditions are comparable. The IOM study identified the provider–patient interaction as a key factor in improving quality of care through such methods as educational interventions to increase cultural competency among providers and referral methods to increase racial concordance between patients and providers. When discussing immigrant nurses, it is important to understand how their role as health care providers may have relevance for health disparities in the US.

In the United States, it has been widely established that racial/ethnic differences between providers and patients affects quality of care, access to care, health care service provision and screening (Geiger, 1996; Cooper and Powe, 2004). The potential barriers to effective interactions between immigrant nurses and their patients can be daunting, ranging from cultural differences – both medical and ethnic – to linguistic, religious and social class differences (Fiscella et al., 1997). The fact that immigrant providers – both nurses and doctors – are recruited to serve in poor, often urban hospitals is significant because such health care settings already have formidable challenges, such as insufficient staff and resources and the complex needs of relatively poor, multiracial and ethnic patient populations that US born and trained health care providers find challenging (Mick, Lee and Wodchis, 2000). While the presence of immigrant providers in urban safety net health facilities could have significant effects, both positive and negative, on the quality of care and health disparities, there is very little research conducted on these issues (Arends-Kunning, 2006).

It is also critical to examine relationships between immigrant health care providers and their American trained co-providers on a medical team. The above-mentioned IOM report identified the work of interdisciplinary teams and teamwork as a potential strategy for improving health outcomes for racial/ethnic minorities. The multi-professional medical team has become a standard goal in American hospitals, especially with the introduction of total patient care approaches in the 1990s and the need for the integration of different professional contributions to patient care in the restructured workplace (McCallan, 2001). For Indian nurses, the differences in professional culture are enormous, particularly in the relationships with their co-providers (nurses, LVNs, physicians). Despite these significant differences, little empirical scholarship exists on these matters.

Nursing Shortages and Immigrant Nurses in the US

In the US, a number of factors have contributed to the increased demand for nurses. The post-World War II expansion of Medicare and Medicaid programmes created a greater need for health care professionals. Economic growth in the 1950s and 1960s allowed more employers to offer medical insurance to their workers. However, the supply of nursing personnel did not maintain pace with the expansion of the demand for health care, leading to cyclical patterns of nursing shortage (Arends-Kuenning, 2006).

One of the main reasons for the shortage was an increase in attractive alternate career choices for women leading to the decline in the traditional labour pool of US born women choosing the nursing profession. Furthermore, sex-based occupational discrimination along with poor working conditions for nurses resulted not only in the shortage of new nurses but also a high exit rate for those already in the profession (Jackson et al., 1989).

The liberalisation of immigration, specifically in the form of the Immigration and Nationality Act of 1965, was an attempt to respond to such labour shortages in the US economy. Because this Act allowed for the entry of skilled professionals who were needed in the US and also increased immigration quotas for formerly restricted areas, it helped induce an increase in immigration of Indian nurses along with other Asian nurses. By the late 1970s, immigration of Indian nurses to the US was only exceeded by that of Filipina nurses and closely followed by Korean nurses. From 1975–1979, while 11.9 per cent of the nurses admitted to the US as permanent residents were from India, 27.6 per cent were from the Philippines and 11.2 per cent were from Korea (Ishi, 1987). In the last US National Sample Survey of Registered Nurses, 38.9 per cent and 10.9 per cent of sampled foreign nurses came from the Philippines and India respectively (Spratley et al., 2000).

Kerala Christian Nurses

The majority of immigrant Indian nurses come from the southern Indian state of Kerala, where the British colonial legacy had initiated the recruitment of young Christian women into the profession of nursing. The initial and relative openness of the Christian communities to nursing had much to do with the active role that English missionaries and mission hospitals took in representing nursing as noble Christian service as opposed to the broader Indian societal perspective that it was a low status profession associated with pollution and impurity (Ragavachari, 1990).

Although the state of Kerala is considered a developmental model for its achievements in areas such as education and health, consistently high unemployment rates have promoted migration of the state's educated young, particularly nurses. Thus Kerala Christian nurses not only supplied India's need for nurses but eventually immigrated to many parts of the world to meet the global demand for nurses. While no accurate figures exist on the population of Indian nurses in the US or of Kerala immigrants, a directory on Keralites in the US indicates that 85 per cent of these immigrants are Christians whereas Christians make up only one fifth of Kerala's population (Andrews, 1983). Scholars attribute the disproportionate presence of Christians among the Keralites in the US to nursing professionals who tend to be from the Christian community (Williams, 1988, 1996).

The story of the Kerala nurses and their immigration is connected to another story about the transformation of women's worth in Kerala. The discourse around the female child in Kerala was one that equated her with a liability. In a society where arranged marriage is still the norm, daughters were often seen as 'burdens', since the family was obliged to provide a dowry for the marriage of daughters. From being burdens and liabilities, the young nurses became transformed into financial assets within the family. As nursing opened up a window of opportunity for young women to earn money and contribute to the family income, there was a concurrent change in their status both in the family and in the wider Kerala society. Their increased earning capacity and independence in their lives became the basis for the societal evaluation of nurses as deviating from respectable gender norms.

For example, I discovered that despite the association with noble Christian service, there was a stigma against nurses as 'loose and dirty' women (George, 2005). I first became alerted to the existence of this stigma in a conversation with a group of immigrant Indian nurses who all got very excited at the chance mention of this stigma by one of them. I learned that the stigma against nursing came from two sources in Kerala. First, nurses were linked with moral looseness because of their close associations with male doctors and patients. In a society where young girls were not allowed to be present in the company of male visitors who were not relatives, to be touching and cleaning the bodies of male patients was scandalous and gave rise to allegations of sexual immorality against nurses as a group. Second, nurses were assumed to be from lower class origins because of the 'menial' nature of the work and the assumption that only poor families with no other means would have let their daughters go into nursing. The social/cultural change that the nursing professional identity brought to these women met different marginalising forces in the US.

Methods

This chapter emerges from a larger qualitative study that examined the gendered immigration and settlement of Indian nurses (George, 2005). Focusing on the three spheres of work, home and community, I conducted 18 months of ethnography in a community of Indian nurses and their families in a metropolitan area of the US and six months of ethnography in the sending community in India to examine the changes in gender relations after immigration in each of the spheres. I used participant-observation methods in an immigrant Indian church and in a nursing home where many nurses worked and interviewed nurses and their husbands in their homes. In India, I interviewed family members of 20 immigrant nurses I had interviewed in the US as well as several deans and professors of nursing schools, retired and active nurses working in India and church leaders to understand the effects of transnational migration on gender relations.

The data for this chapter comes from 24 in-depth semi-structured interviews lasting an hour to two hours with immigrant Indian nurses working in a US metropolitan area. The interviews were conducted in the language of the participant's choice (English or Malayalam, and sometimes a mix) and in the venue of the participant's choice (mostly in the nurses' homes or workplaces). The interview domains included general questions about decision to go into nursing, incentives and processes of migration, educational and work experiences in India and the US. Ethical approval for the project was granted from the Institutional Review Board of the University of California, Berkeley. Ethnography in the US immigrant church and involvement in community programmes allowed for the use of a convenience sampling approach to interview participant selection. The nurses interviewed were all women and married with the exception of one widow. The findings of this study display a consistent level of uniformity among those interviewed.

Although it was culturally inappropriate to ask their ages directly, the participants' ages at time of interview was estimated by using the date by which they finished high school. The mean age of the participants at the time of their interview was estimated to be 44 years with a standard deviation of 3.7 years. The years of initial migration for the women from their villages to nursing schools within India ranged from 1963 to 1979 (mean of 1968) with a standard deviation of 3.7 years. The year of arrival in the United States ranged from 1971 to 1991 (mean of 1977) with a standard deviation of 4.3 years. The occupational level at the time of interview was highly similar with 19 participants being RNs and four participants working at higher or lower levels. Sixteen of those interviewed reported that they immigrated to the US exclusively on their own volition whereas six reported either partially shared or fully delegated decision-making.

I translated the interviews and transcribed them verbatim soon after they had taken place, allocating pseudonyms to each participant to ensure confidentiality. The transcription process and several readings of the transcripts thereafter along with triangulation with field notes from participant observation allowed me to develop a holistic sense for the experiences described by the participants. The transcripts of the data were coded and indexed to develop analytical categories and theoretical explanations within and across interviews. These categories were derived inductively, using an open coding process and hypotheses were organically developed from the ground up (Patton, 2002).

Results

The nurses I interviewed told me that while they had heard about the difficulties of obtaining work permits and licenses, they were unprepared for the challenging interactions with patients, co-providers and hospital administrators, the different social organisation of the work place and the distinct professional standards of nursing in the US.

Challenging Social Interactions

Many of the nurses spoke of their experiences of being rejected by patients who openly asked for 'white nurses' or suggested, '[w]hy don't you go back to your country?' A finding that is also reflected in the literature on foreign nurses (Xu, 2005; Allan et al., 2004; Taylor, 2005). One of the nurses I interviewed, Mrs Eapen,[2] worked on a floor where she and two other immigrant nurses covered the weekend evening shifts. She described an incident where a patient expressed his lack of faith in her professional capacity:

> So he (the patient) said, 'I want to see a nurse'. We both had uniforms on. We both had our identification badges. So I said 'We are nurses. My name is Susie and this is Nanny. We are both registered nurses'. He said, 'I want to see a real nurse'. So I said, 'We have our registration. We are registered nurses. So I think we are real nurses'.

Other nurses talked about the difficulties of working with a patient population with diverse social and medical problems, particularly in urban publicly funded facilities. For example, Mrs Thomas noted:

> Maybe the other hospitals are different. (In) County hospitals, you are not paid well. IV-drug patients, all these alcoholic patients, patients living immoral lives – so many are in the county hospital. Not all the people – some are angry with us. We don't take it personally. We take abuse from the patients. That is our job, (to take) verbal abuse from the patients. In the county, everybody is equal. Nobody can say anything.

The challenges of social interaction with co-providers for the Indian immigrant nurses ranged from being distrusted to being ignored to having difficulty with social banter. Some nurses told me that they felt surveiled by their co-providers who appeared to be checking up on them behind their backs. Other nurses spoke

---

2   While recognising that both race and ethnicity are socially constructed categories, I use both terms together to cover the range of biological and social variables associated with them and to highlight their common role in stereotyping social groups through biological reductionism and cultural essentialism (Oppenheimer, 2001).

of instances where doctors passed them by to ask American-trained colleagues questions about the immigrant nurses' own patients. Mrs Eapen talked about just such encounters as follows:

> Doctors they – some of them, they see you – they don't ask you anything because they think you don't know anything. The residents are pretty good but some attendings – they don't ask you, they go and ask another white nurse and she will say, 'It's not my patient. It's so and so's patient'. Then he (the doctor), even though he passed you by, he comes back to ask you about your patient. Then you think 'Why did he pass me by? Why didn't he ask me first and see whose patient that was?' ... But not now. I mean, now I can't see that happening because I've been there for a long time.

Mrs Eapen's experience of being ignored by physicians may have been the result of being new to the hospital as much as due to her immigrant status since she now feels that as a seasoned veteran of the hospital, it would be unlikely that co-providers would ignore her.

One immediate problem for the immigrant nurses was their lack of cultural capital, which made it difficult to for them to interact socially with their peers. Despite not having a 'language problem', Mrs Philip explained why she was having difficulty at work when she said:

> It takes courage to be with people and talk and laugh and joke like they are doing. I still feel the difference being with white people, because I don't even understand them. Maybe it is my age difference with the group. Although they are at work, they talk about life at home, like their boyfriends and girlfriends, stuff like that, where I can't talk in that way with them.

In addition to dealing with patients and co-providers, the immigrant nurses also had to contend with career advancement issues and what they reported as differential treatment from managers and administrators, a finding that is also reported by researchers in the UK (Alexis and Vydelingum, 2004; Allan et al., 2004). Mrs Lukos talked about the discrepancy of treatment that she received from a nurse manager regarding a test that was required for all the employees in the intensive care unit where she worked. The nurse manager singled Mrs Lukos out with the forewarning that she could not work in that unit if she did not pass the test. Mrs Lukos found out that none of her American colleagues had received similar warnings. She surmised that she had been given the special treatment because '[t]he nurse manager thought I am from a foreign country and I am not intelligent enough to pass'. While Mrs Lukos passed with a high grade of 98 per cent she found out that one of her American colleagues had failed the test and was still scheduled to work. She challenged the nurse manager's double standards successfully and the American nurse could not continue working in that unit.

Occupational Mobility and Immobility

Whether working as nurses' aides, licensed registered nurses or attempting to rise up to managerial levels, the Indian immigrant nurses had to work within a complex system, making occupational mobility challenging.

Because of the difficulty and time involved in passing the state boards, most foreign nurses, working with other mostly minority women, obtained jobs as nurses' aides in the meantime to make ends meet. Some states granted an interim permit for those foreign educated nurses who had met the prerequisites to take the next scheduled RN licensing exam; however, in most states, the only professional option for unlicensed nurses was to work as nurses' aides. Without passing the state boards, they tended to work as nurses' aides with other mostly minority women.

Many of the nurses I interviewed found it very hard to work as nurses' aides for a number of reasons. It was emotionally difficult to do work that they believed had little to do with nursing. For example, several of the Indian nurses recalled that there were 'ayahs' or 'methranis' in Indian hospitals – women with no professional education – who emptied bed pans and cleaned up after incontinent patients. In India, this kind of 'direct nursing work' – the dirty work – was left to nursing students, family members and ayahs. For women like Mrs Punoose it was a shock to find out that in America, even 'the nursing director will do the work of a nurse if it is necessary'. Scholarship on immigrant nurses shows that after immigration, not only must they readjust to a new philosophy about the different types of labour that are included within the professional duties of nursing (Xu, 2005), but they must also face a demotion of their professional status and a discrediting of their past experience as staff nurses when they become nurses' aides (Allan and Larsen, 2003; Taylor, 2005).

Working as nurses' aides, many immigrant nurses ended up performing the work of registered nurses while getting paid aides' salaries (Sexton, 1981). Mrs Eapen explained how this came about in her case as follows:

> I knew what to do. I knew how to change dressings. I studied in India plus when the IV bottles were empty I could change the IV solution for them if they were at lunch or they were busy. The things that I was not supposed to do as a nursing assistant, I was doing for the nurses. Either they asked me or I just had the free time and I used to do it.

For those who passed the exam, getting a job was not very difficult given the shortage in nursing. With licenses in hand, not only were they more likely to be recruited for inner-city hospitals with other mostly Asian immigrant nurses, but they were also more likely to work in wards that were physically labour intensive and in areas with a high burnout rate for US trained nurses (Ong and Azores, 1994; Arends Kuenning, 2006). Once licensed, immigrant nurses tend to work for more years than US-trained nurses who experience burn-out and leave the profession earlier (Arends Kuenning, 2006; Xu, 2006). And even in these least sought after jobs, Indian nurses reported discrimination in the lack of appreciation and equal wages as recounted by Mrs Samuel:

> ... In some places, you feel depressed. Same job, same amount of work, same thing you do, and still they appreciate the whites. Whatever the whites do, they will bring it up. We are doing the same job – passed the same exam, but they still pay them (white nurses) more.

There is some evidence in the literature that immigrant nurses may suffer wage discrimination. For example, the US Equal Employment Opportunity Commission (EEOC) settled a class employment discrimination lawsuit for $2.1 million dollars against a US health care centre which was found to have discriminated against 65 Filipino nurses by paying them $6/hour less than their US trained counterparts (EEOC, 1999).

And even though immigrant nurses have long careers as nurses, few rise to management level leadership positions. A recent study in the US reports that from 1977 to 2000, both proportions of immigrant nurses in management and their work time in supervisory functions dropped markedly (Xu and Kwak, 2006). Part of the reason for this maybe that there are barriers of discrimination – such as lack of appreciation for their efforts, as compared to white colleagues (DiCicco-Bloom, 2004; Allan and Larsen, 2003). Mrs Lukos, a nurse manager, was an exception among those women I interviewed because she was a nurse manager, yet she spoke about the difficulties of her position as follows:

> I have to do fifteen times more than what a white person does to survive as a manager. And my opportunities are also fifteen times less. ... In order to get the next promotion as a Vice President of nursing I have to work fifteen times more. That's the system.

On the other hand, many nurses were not in a position to focus on career advancement, given their family obligations. Because they were not only supporting themselves and their immediate families but also extended family in India, the nurses I interviewed tended to work long and hard hours and use many strategies to earn higher incomes. Consequently, most of the immigrant nurses, who were already stretched for time, were not interested in additional managerial responsibilities with minimal extra compensation.

The literature suggests that racism may play a part in the relative lack of career mobility for immigrant and minority nurses (Allan et al., 2004; Winkelmann-Gleed, 2006). However, it is important to acknowledge that this is a complicated issue since it is not always easy to assess claims that racism directly and exclusively hinders career progression. Winkelmann-Gleed points out that while the marked imbalance in the racial makeup of the managerial component as compared to the general staff in British National Health Services raises questions about the fairness of the promotion processes, '[t]here are complex reasons why individuals do not progress, are unable to progress or do not wish to progress in their careers' (2006, p. 81).

Differences in Professional Skills and Values: 'Real Nursing Work' versus
'Charting and Sweet Talking'

In the face of the devaluation of their work and the social segregation of the ward floor, the immigrant nurses I interviewed resisted by defining the work they did as 'real nursing work' as compared to the nursing done by American nurses. The distinction goes as follows: Indian nurses are better at doing the 'actual' work of nursing – the practical work of bandaging patients, checking IVs and inserting catheters; whereas, American nurses are good at 'charting, writing and sweet talking'.

A number of the immigrant nurses, like Mrs Simon, complained about how American nurses get away with not doing the 'real nursing work'. As she put it:

> I see – like a couple of nurses, not everybody – just a couple of nurses – they come and they sit and they talk, talk, and talk. But you hardly see them moving around and working – I mean the real nursing job.

> Are these immigrant nurses? [George]

> No, these are white Americans. They will flirt around with white doctors – Bah, bah, bah, bah – I mean, we don't go for all these things. We come, do our job, take care of our patients, say 'Hi, I am so and so' and we do our job. The Americans have a way of saying – 'Hi honey, how are you? Hi sweetheart'. I mean, I have even seen nurses kissing the patients. We don't go for all that. And the patient likes that – the patient thinks 'Oh, the nurse – so wonderful she is'. You know what I mean? Those nurses can act a lot. They get better feedback from patients. At the same time, we may be working hard and we may not be getting that much appreciation.

In Mrs Simon's eyes, the American nurses can do less 'real nursing work' because they are good at sweet-talking the patients and flirting with the doctors. While Mrs Simon characterises her partiality to 'real nursing work' as a choice – 'We don't go for all these things' – it seems likely that Mrs Simon would be less successful at kissing the patients and flirting with the white doctors. Thus, Mrs Simon and her ilk may be limited to doing what she calls 'real nursing work'.

Secondly, Mrs Simon counterpoised 'real nursing work' with 'paperwork', which she characterised as preferred by white nurses. She talked about the ambulatory unit – where patients report before surgery – as made up of all white nurses who mostly do paperwork. Because the patients in the ambulatory unit are not yet bedridden, they do not require much practical nursing care. Mrs Simon described her reticence to work in ambulatory nursing as follows:

I don't like ambulatory nursing because it's not really nursing – it's like more of an office nurse type. Lot of paperwork – I really don't like doing paperwork much. I like to do real nursing. You know it's stimulating – watching the blood pressure and checking the patient's fluid levels – things like that are more like nursing to me. Ambulatory (nursing) could be boring sometimes. Sometimes it could be so busy that it could make you confused if you are not used to it. All the patients come and so many people you have to send together to the OR (Operating Room). You have to check everybody. You have to be careful – anything you didn't do and they will call you. So originally the nurses were all white – in ambulatory, they are all white.

At first, Mrs Simon identifies her distaste for working in the ambulatory unit as a choice. She prefers to do 'real nursing', which is more stimulating than paperwork but she then admits that doing all the paperwork in the ambulatory unit could be confusing for her. Consequently, she and other nurses like herself may end up in wards that are physically more labour intensive with less paperwork.

The literature points to differences between sending and host countries in professional expectations of immigrant nurses, leading to a lack of fit between the nurses' nursing values and skills and those of the health care organisations they serve after immigration (Matiti and Taylor, 2005; Xu, 2005; 2006). Consequently 'the real nursing work' as described by my study participants – the practical skills of nursing – may have been more highly valued in the Indian healthcare contexts as opposed to an increased emphasis after migration on the management of paperwork and relationships with patients and co-workers in multidisciplinary teams (Allan and Larsen, 2003: Xu, 2005; 2006; Matiti and Taylor, 2005).

For example, 'total patient care' was identified as a nursing practice that was different from what they were accustomed to in India by several of my study participants. As Mrs Thomas explained:

… Here nursing is about total patient care, the total wellbeing of the patient – mental and physical care of the patient as well as the patient's family. Back home you give medicines, that is all.

Several nurses emphasised the new role of teaching since US law requires that patients are made aware of the effects of each medication and medical procedure and it is primarily the duty of the nurse to keep patients informed, to question doctors and pharmacists in case of mistakes regarding the appropriate medications and dosages (Xu, 2006; Taylor, 2005). While immigrant nurses are practicing their profession in new and varied ways as patient care managers and teachers, they may struggle with reconciling the skills and values they bring with them with the different requirements in their new work settings.

Discussion

It is well established by sociologists that the labour market in the United States is stratified by various socially-based divisions such as race and gender, which results in particular types of workers being segregated into labour sectors with unequal pay and less access to opportunities for advancement. That many lower paying, lower status jobs are mostly populated by minority women, reflects how the interlocking nature of race and gender shapes the division of labour in society (Nakanno Glenn, 1992; Roberts, 1997).

Nursing as a profession is gendered, in that women are stereotypically seen as ideal candidates because of their 'essential' psychological tendencies to be nurturing, self-sacrificing and subordinate (Soothill and Kendrick, 1992). Furthermore, the division of labour in nursing is racialised because minority and immigrant nurses are often found in low status jobs, positioned on the lower rungs of the nursing professional hierarchy (nursing aides and licensed vocational nurses below registered nurses) (Sexton, 1981; Glazer, 1988). When recruited to positions higher in the professional hierarchy, they tend to work in relatively lower paying, inner-city health care settings and in wards with high burn-out rates for white and US trained nurses (for example, ICUs and other critical care wards) (Sexton, 1981; Glazer, 1991; DiCicco-Bloom, 2004). The Indian immigrant nurses I interviewed also seemed to be referring to such a racialised division of labour.

A racialised division of labour and a distinct professional hierarchy map over each other to create a grid – a racialised hierarchy – which may limit the immigrant nurses' professional mobility in the United States. The Indian immigrant nurses' experiences of antagonism in their social interactions with patients, co-providers and administrators suggest the existence of such a racialised hierarchy. The notions of 'real nurses' and 'real nursing work' seem to also point to the existence of such a hierarchy within the nursing profession. Similarly Allan and colleagues (2004) found that the hierarchical nature of British nursing and the grading system were the cause for institutional racism and discrimination against immigrant nurses in the UK. The immigrant nurses I interviewed, who on one hand have attained hard-won US credentials (their RN licenses) to become 'real nurses' and who experience their work as 'real nursing work' (the practical work of changing IVs, monitoring patient's symptoms and other technical tasks), are assessed as 'not real' nurses by patients, seemingly distrusted by co-providers, under appreciated by administration and limited in their career mobility within the system.

This analysis suggests four general factors that contribute to the racialised hierarchy in the urban nursing working environment within which the Indian immigrant nurses I interviewed found themselves doing more physically intensive 'real nursing work' instead of 'charting, writing and sweet talking'. They include: 1) the racialisation of the Indian nurses; 2) the general distrust of foreigners in the immigrant nurses' urban work environments; 3) the gendered and racialised expectation of emotional labour within nursing, which the Indian nurses are less likely to meet; and 4) the pre-migration work experiences that the nurses bring from India, including distinct professional and ethnic cultural dimensions, which shape their US work experiences, preferences and opportunities.

The racialisation of the immigrant nurses after immigration is a key factor that affects their experiences in the work place. By racialisation, I follow Omi and Winant's definition to mean 'an extension of racial meaning to a previously racially unclassified relationship, social practice or group' (Omi and Winant, 1989, p. 64). Consequently, the Indian nurses, who prior to immigration have no experience of being a racial/ethnic minority, become minorities in the United States as they are placed into a racial/ethnic category about which they know little. All the nurses I interviewed had been given no orientation to the social and political history of the United States and found themselves manoeuvring their way around new American social categories of race/ethnicity in their work places without much guidance.

Urban hospitals, with a mix of racial/ethnic groups, presented racially charged environments where the Indian nurses were left to sink or swim. For example, there is a great deal of evidence in the literature that African Americans, who make up a primary segment of the US urban safety-net hospital populations, tend to distrust the medical establishment because of a legacy of racial discrimination and the violation of human rights in medical research and the health care system (Bryd and Clayton, 2000). Given the historical medical injustices experienced by African Americans, it is feasible that the disproportionate presence of immigrant nurses in urban hospitals may have been interpreted as evidence of a lower quality of care being offered to minorities. Consequently, the verbal abuse and rejection by patients in urban county hospital settings described by the Indian immigrant nurses may be partially explained by such factors.

The literature on minority and immigrant nurses suggests that such nurses feel isolated, frustrated, exploited and angry because of racism from patients as well as staff and management (Allan and Larsen, 2003; Allan et al., 2004; Alexis and Vydelingum, 2004; DiCicco-Bloom, 2004). Allan et al. (2004), following Goldberg (1993), argue that because of its contextual and fluid nature, racism is hard to prove from the oppressed person's point of view. They cite the example of a participant in their study who is not sure whether she was not given a certain job because she was 'overqualified' or because she was a black African woman.

A second factor is the general distrust of foreigners – on account of such differences as related to language, accent, skin colour and culture – which may have contributed to a questioning of the professional competency of the nurses and led to distrust on the part of patients, co-providers and managers. Interpreting discrimination can be challenging as there seems to be a component of discrimination that may have to do with the foreign background and different culture of immigrant nurses (Allan et al., 2004; Taylor, 2005). Literature from the UK suggests that white overseas nurses can experience discrimination based on the 'foreign' factor (Allan et al., 2004; Taylor, 2005). With foreignness comes the questioning of qualifications and credentials and the implication that nurses from other countries may bring down the professional nursing standards of the host country (Joel, 1996). Yet US census data shows that immigrant nurses have higher educational levels than their US born counterparts and the technical qualifications necessary to do the job (Ahrends Kuenning, 2006). Nevertheless, it may have been the 'foreign' factor that explains some of the reasons why some patients openly rejected these nurses and asked for 'real nurses' and why co-providers appeared to distrust and surveil their international colleagues and why administrators seemed to utilise different standards for the promotion of immigrant nurses as compared to their American colleagues.

A third factor is the gendered expectation of emotional labour within nursing work, which was difficult for the Indian nurses to meet. Sociologist Arlie Hochschild defines emotional labour as 'the management of feeling to create a publicly observable facial and bodily display [which] is sold for a wage and therefore has exchange value' (Hochschild, 1983, p. 6). Nursing is often identified as the archetypal feminised profession that involves a great deal of emotional labour (Mann, 2005; Bolton, 2001). Yet, while the physical rigours of patient care or working in the health care setting are clearly identified, the emotional demands for nurses are commonly overlooked and not explicitly stated in a nursing job description nor fully appreciated as part of the nurse's labour (Smith and Gray, 2000). It is argued that the under appreciation of emotional labour in professions such as nursing reflects an overall devaluation of care work – the labour of providing care, including its fundamentally emotional components, for a wage – at a societal level (Cancian and Oliker, 2000; Stone, 2000).

Even though care work and its emotional dimensions maybe under valued at a societal level, it appears that not all women's care work is equally undervalued. For example, feminist scholarship points to the racialised occupational segregation within care work, where women of colour are often relegated to the less desirable menial, manual 'dirty, back rooms' (for example, maids, house cleaners) whereas white women are concentrated in the jobs requiring the most relational interaction and wear the public face of care work (Nakano Glenn, 1992; Roberts, 1997). Furthermore, it is argued that an examination of the racial/ethnic hierarchies within care work not only points to the concentration of white women in jobs that have strong relational and emotional components but also to the better paying and more professionalised nature of these jobs compared to their less emotionally labour-intensive counterparts (Nakano Glenn, 1992; Roberts, 1997).

Mrs Simon and other Indian nurses found similar gendered expectations of emotional labour within the hospital wards where they worked. That white nurses 'kissed the patients and flirted with the doctors' and were concentrated in the ambulatory and recovery units (relatively less physically labour intensive, better paid and higher status units) while Mrs Simon and her immigrant peers did the physically demanding 'real nursing work' parallels the racialised occupational segregation identified above. Yet the racialised hierarchy in the US was not the only reason why Mrs Simon and other Indian immigrant nurses were, for the most part, segregated in the 'back rooms' of the urban, safety-net hospitals and in the most physically labour intensive units.

Rather, and this being a fourth factor that solidified their position in the grid, their work experiences and the professional and ethnic cultures that they brought from India also contributed to their choice to do 'real nursing work'. What was an especially revealing insight from my research was that the main point of reference for the Indian immigrant nurses was their work experiences in India, which were shaped by both distinct professional and ethnic cultures specific to their region of India. Whereas the Indian immigrant nurses have professional skills and values that arise out of the specific structural and cultural conditions of their nursing training and practice contexts, these skills and values may not be congruent within the new health care contexts where they find themselves after migration.

The professional culture of nursing in India had developed from different structural conditions of the Indian health care system as compared to the United States. For instance, because of the shortage of health care workers, the health provider-to-patient ratio was very large (several nurses reported the ratio of 1 nurse to 45 or 50 patients) relative to the one they encountered in the United States (for example, State of California requires a ratio of 1 nurse to 5 patients). Several nurses pointed out that the larger nurse-to-patient ratio in India made it very difficult to know or interact with patients on a personal basis. Also, family members were typically present with patients in Indian hospitals and took care of their non-medical needs, perhaps due to the shortage of health care workers as is true in other resource poor countries (Xu, 2005; Matiti and Taylor, 2005). Consequently, the Indian immigrant nurses I interviewed reported not having to interact extensively with their Indian patients and know them personally as they were expected to do in the US.

There were several aspects of the Indian ethnic culture that affected the nurses' inability to successfully meet the different standards of emotional caring in the US work setting. Public expression of closeness and emotional intimacy in formal relationships are not consonant with wider Indian cultural norms, similar to many Asian cultures. However, such expression is not only more consistent with the norms in wider American culture but expected as part of nursing care by patients, co-workers and family members and is also part of the measure of high quality care.

The nurses I interviewed were also less comfortable with such expression, given the Indian gender norms that constrain such behaviours in public, even for married couples. Furthermore, as nurses from Kerala, India, they had been trained and developed their professional behaviour under the shadow of regional gender-based stigmas that associated sexual looseness and immorality with all nurses because they associated so closely with male doctors and patients (George, 2005). Consequently, it was not surprising to hear the Indian immigrant nurses I interviewed express discomfort at their perception that such physical displays of affection were required of them to be seen as good nurses. That is, many of them were not comfortable doing 'emotional labour' or at least to the extent displayed by some of their American-trained colleagues in the United States. In sum, besides the limitations placed on them by the racialised hierarchy in the US nursing context, their work experiences, preferences and opportunities may have been shaped also by the particular professional skills and cultural values that they brought with them.

Conclusion

With the ongoing nursing shortage and the continuing recruitment of immigrant nurses, it is important to recognise that they may face a number of challenges to incorporation in their new work settings. The findings of this study point to four factors: 1) racialisation in the US work environments; 2) distrust of foreigners and consequent negative relationships with patients, co-providers and administrators; 3) gendered and racialised expectations of emotional labour in nursing; and 4) the impact of pre-migration Indian work experiences and training, shaped by unique ethnic and professional cultures. The different professional expectations in the United States along with difficult work environments, including rejection by patients, the seeming distrust of co-providers and under appreciation administration, increased the level of tension for the Indian immigrant nurses I interviewed. These burdens could likely place limits on these workers' ability to function effectively with co-providers in team efforts. How they navigate through their new work environments and respond to the differing professional expectations may have implication for the quality of care that they are perceived as providing and potentially for health disparities among the patients they serve.

Quality of care is an important issue for patients in US inner city health care settings that has repercussions vis-à-vis health disparities in this population (Cooper and Powe, 2004). Research shows that if such patients perceive that the quality of care is compromised, they may access care late, not follow medical advice and refuse screening for diseases (Blanchard and Lurie, 2004). For immigrant nurses to be better positioned to serve their patients, particularly in US urban, underserved hospitals, they could be more actively integrated into their work settings through appropriate orientation programmes that specifically address the historical, political and sociological aspects of US race and ethnic relations and the different professional standards and ethnic cultural norms in such settings.

Currently, there are no standardardised induction programmes that introduce immigrant nurses in the US to their work settings. Patients, US trained medical staff and administrators could be better informed about the backgrounds and qualifications of international recruits as well. Additional research needs to be conducted at the point of delivery of care to further understand the specific ways in which a racialised division of labour in society and a professional hierarchy within nursing come together with the particular professional skill and values brought by immigrant nurses to shape the experiences, preferences and opportunities of these nurses and potentially impact quality of care for underserved populations.

References

Aiken, L., Buchan, J., Sochalski, J., Nichols, B. and Powell, M., 2004. Trends in International Nurse Migration, *Health Affairs*, 23(3), pp. 69–77.

Alexis, O. and Vydelingum, V., 2004. The Lived Experience of Overseas Black and Minority Ethnic Nurses in the NHS in the South of England. *Diversity in Health and Social Care*, 1(1), pp. 13–20.

Allan, H.T. and Larsen, J.A., 2003. 'We Need Respect': Experiences of internationally recruited nurses in the UK. Available through University of Surrey, European Institute of Health and Medical Sciences: <http://www.rcn. org.uk/downloads/international/irn-report-we-need-respect.pdf> [Accessed 24 April 2006].

Allan, H.T, Larsen, J.A., Bryan, K. and Smith, P., 2004. The Social Reproduction of Institutional Racism: Internationally recruited nurses' experiences of the British health services. *Diversity in Health and Social Care*, 1(2), pp. 117–25.

Andrews, K.P., 1983. *Keralites in AMERICA: Community reference book.* New York: Literary Market Review Inc.

Arends-Kuenning, M., 2006. The Balance of Care: Trends in the wages and employment of immigrant nurses in the US between 1990 and 2000. *Globalizations*, 3(9), pp. 333–48.

Blanchard, J. and Lurie, N., 2004. R-E-S-P-E-C-T: Patient reports of disrespect in health care setting and its impact on care. *The Journal of Family Practice*, 53(9), pp. 721–30.

Bolton, S.C., 2001. Changing Faces: Nurses as emotional jugglers. *Sociology of Health and Illness*, 23(1), pp. 85–100.

Bryd, W. and Clayton, L., 2000. *An American Health Dilemma: A medical history of African Americans and the problem of race.* New York: Routledge.

Cancian, F.M. and Oliker, S.J., 2000. *Caring and Gender.* Thousand Oaks, CA: Pine Forge Press.

Charmaz, K., 1994. 'Discovering' Chronic Illness: Using grounded theory. In: B.G. Glaser, ed. 1994. *More Grounded Theory Methodology: A reader.* Mill Valley, CA: Sociology Press. pp. 65–94.

Cooper, L. and Powe, N., 2004. Disparities in Patient Experiences, Health Care Processes, and Outcomes: The role of patient-provider racial, ethnic and language concordance. [online] Available through Commonwealth Fund website: <http://www.commonwealthfund.org/Publications/Fund-Reports/2004/Jul/Disparities-in-Patient-Experiences--Health-Care-Processes--and-Outcomes--The-Role-of-Patient-Provide.aspx> [Accessed on 24 April 2007].

Curran, C.R., Minnick, A. and Moss, J., 1987. Who Needs Nurses? *American Journal of Nursing*, (April), p. 444.

DiCicco-Bloom, B., 2004. The Racial and Gendered Experiences of Immigrant Nurses from Kerala, India. *Journal of Transcultural Nursing*, 15(1), pp. 26–33.

Fiscella, K., Roman-Diaz, M., Lue, B., Botelho, R. and Frankel, R., 1997. 'Being a Foreigner, I May Be Punished if I Make a Small Mistake': Assessing transcultural experiences in caring for patients. *Family Practice*, 14(2), pp. 112–16.

Geiger, H.J., 1996. Race and Health Care: An American dilemma? *New England Journal of Medicine*, 335(11), pp. 815–16.

George, S., 2005. *When Women Come First: Gender and class in transnational migration*. Berkeley, CA: University of California Press.

Glazer, N.Y., 1991. 'Between a rock and a hard place': Women's professional organizations in nursing and class, racial, and ethnic inequalities. *Gender and Society*, 5(3), pp. 351–72.

Hochschild, A.R., 1983. *The Managed Heart: Commercialization of human feeling*. Berkeley, CA: University of California Press.

Ishi, T., 1987. Class Conflict, the State and Linkage: The international migration of nurses from the Philippines. *Berkeley Journal of Sociology*, 32, pp. 281–312.

Jackson, J., MacFalda, P.A. and McManus, K., 1989. Status of the Nursing Shortage and Projections. In: T.F. Moore and E.A. Simendinger, eds. 1989. *Managing the Nursing Shortage: A guide to recruitment and retention*. Rockville, Md: Aspen Publishers. pp. 264–70.

Joel, L. 1996. Immigration: Why is It Still up for Discussion? *American Journal of Nursing*, 96(1), p. 7.

Mann, S., 2005. A Health-Care Model of Emotional Labor: An evaluation of the literature and development of a model. *Journal of Health Organization and Management*, 19(4/5), pp. 304–17.

Matiti, M.R. and Taylor, D., 2005. The Cultural Lived Experience of Internationally Recruited Nurses: A phenomenological study. *Diversity in Health and Social Care*, 2(1), pp. 7–16.

McCallan, A., 2001. Interdisciplinary Practice – A matter of teamwork: An integrated literature review. *Journal of Clinical Nursing*, 10(4), pp. 419–28.

Mejia, A., Pizurki, H. and Royston, E., 1979. *Physician and Nurse Migration: Analysis and policy implications*. Geneva: World Health Organization.

Mick, S.S., Lee, S.D. and Wodchis, W.P., 2000. Variations in the Distribution of Foreign and Domestically Trained Physicians in the United States: 'Safety net' or 'surplus exacerbation'? *Social Science and Medicine*, 50(2), pp. 185–202.

Nakano Glenn, E., 1992. From Servitude to Service Work: Historical continuities in the racial division of paid reproductive labor. *Signs: Journal of Women in Culture and Society*, 18(1), pp. 1–43.

Omi, M. and Winant, H., 1989. *Racial Formation in the United States: From the 1960s to the 1980s*. New York: Routledge Press.

Ong, P., and Azores, T., 1994. The Migration and Incorporation of Filipino Nurses. In: P. Ong, E. Bonacich and L. Cheng, eds. 1994. *The New Asian Immigration in Los Angeles and Global Restructuring*. Philadelphia, PA: Temple University Press, pp. 164–95.

Oppenheimer, G.M., 2001. Paradigm Lost: Race, ethnicity, and the search for a new population taxonomy. *American Journal of Public Health*, 91(7), 1,049–55.

Patton, M.Q. 2002. *Qualitativer Research and Evaluation Methods.* Thousand Oaks: Sage.

Ragavachari, R., 1990. *Conflicts and Adjustments: Indian nurses in an urban milieu.* Delhi: Academic Foundation.

Redfoot, D.L. and Houser, A.N., 2005. *We Shall Travel On: Quality of care, economic development, and the international migration of long-term care workers.* Washington, DC: AARP Public Policy Institute. Available through AARP website: http://assets.aarp.org/rgcenter/il/2005_14_intl_ltc.pdf [Accessed 24 April 2006].

Roberts, D., 1997. Spiritual and Menial Housework. *Yale Journal of Law and Feminism*, 9, pp. 51–80.

Sexton, P., 1981. *The New Nightingale.* New York: Enquiry.

Smedley, B.D., Stith, A.Y. and Nelson, A.R., eds., 2003. *Unequal Treatment, Confronting Racial and Ethnic Disparities in Health Care.* Washington, DC: National Academies Press.

Soothill, K., Henry, C. and Kendrick, K., eds., 1992. *Themes and Perspectives in Nursing.* New York: Chapman and Hall.

Spratley, E., Johnson, A., Sochalski, J., Fristz, M. and Spencer, W., 2000. *The Registered Nurse Population.* Rockville, MD: Health Resources and Services Administration.

Stone, D., 2000. Why We Need a Care Movement. *The Nation*, 13 March.

Taylor, B., 2005. The Experiences of Overseas Nurses Working in the NHS: Results of a qualitative study. *Diversity in Health and Social Care*, 2(1), pp. 17–28.

The US Equal Employment Opportunity Commission, 1999. *EEOC Announces $2.1 million Settlement of Wage Discrimination Suit for Class of Filipino Nurses.* [online] Available at: <http://www.eeoc.gov/press/3-2-99.html> [Accessed 24 April 2006].

Toro-Morn, M. and Alicea, M., eds., 2004. *Migration and Immigration: A global view.* Westport, CT: Greenwood Press.

Williams, R.B., 1988. *Religions of Immigrants from India and Pakistan: New threads in the American tapestry.* Cambridge: Cambridge University Press.

———, 1996. *Christian Pluralism in the U.S.: The Indian immigrant experience.* Cambridge: Cambridge University Press.

Winkelmann-Gleed, A., 2006. *Migrant Nurses: Motivation, integration and contribution.* Oxford: Radcliffe Publishing.

Xu,Y., 2005. Clinical Challenges of Asian Nurses in a Foreign Health Care Environment. *Home Health Care Management and Practice*, 17(6), pp. 492–4.

———, 2006. Clinical Differences in Nursing between East and West: Implications for Asian nurses. *Home Health Care Management and Practice*, 18(5), pp. 420–23.

Xu, Y. and Kwak, C., 2006. Trended Profile of Internationally Educated Nurses in the United States: Implications for the nurse shortage and beyond. *Journal of Nursing Administration*, 36(11), pp. 522–5.

Chapter 9

Nurses Across Borders: The International Migration of Health Professionals

Stephen Bach

Introduction

It has become widely acknowledged that the international mobility of health professionals provides further evidence of the globalisation of labour markets. Health sector employers especially in English-speaking countries, such as the United States and the United Kingdom, have a long history of recruiting overseas trained health professionals. This reliance has increased over recent decades and there has been increased diversity in source countries (OECD, 2007). In a context of closer global connections between nation states, new actors and institutions have emerged that have re-shaped these global flows and the conditions under which they occur. An emphasis on global circulation is important in highlighting that the health workforce transcends national boundaries, but to unravel the contours and consequences of this mobility necessitates more detailed attention to the behaviour of actors and the influence of institutional rules.

In the past migration specialists have often expressed scepticism about the capacity of government agencies and nation states to influence and control migration flows, especially irregular migration (Castles, 2004). This observation, however, has not precluded attempts to analyse the role of the state as a switching mechanism that can 'change the course of the train, or derail it altogether' (Hollifield, 2008, p. 196). This observation is especially pertinent in a sector like health associated with a high level of state and supra-state intervention and the employment of a large number of professional staff with transferable qualifications. The role of the state in the health sector is accentuated by government influence over the funding of health care provision, its role in establishing service standards for providers that may include staffing levels, and its responsibility for workforce planning and training, to ensure adequate staffing.

Between 2000 and 2009, health care expenditure accounted for a larger proportion of GDP in OECD countries (OECD, 2012). The economic crisis arrested this trend and reinforced an emphasis on cost containment and restructuring, but it has not reversed longer term trends that are increasing the demand for health services. Advances in technology and the availability of new drug therapies are contributing to increased longevity. But an ageing population has also increased the proportion of people that live with chronic long-term health conditions and is reducing the relative size of the working age population. The feminisation of the health professional workforce with more part-time working and the transposition of the EU Working Time Directive, limiting maximum working hours, has also required alterations in working practices and the need to increase workforce capacity (Young, 2011). These trends have already posed significant challenges for governments in ensuring an adequate supply of health professionals and shortages have emerged in most European countries and many other countries in Asia, Australia, the Gulf States and North America. In response to shortages, health systems have become increasingly dependent on the international mobility of health professionals, with employers, often encouraged by government, actively recruiting foreign trained nurses, doctors and other health professionals (OECD, 2007).

The international migration of health professionals in conjunction with shortages has heightened concerns about the global misdistribution of the health workforce and the impact such imbalances have on the health systems of both developing and developed countries. Concerns about 'brain drain', the flow of health professionals from low or middle income countries to high income countries, was prevalent in the 1970s but it was viewed as an 'unpredictable and largely uncontrolled movement' that was 'not a universal phenomenon in that only relatively few countries are heavy donors of physicians and/or nurses, and even fewer are recipients' (Mejia, 1978, p. 207). At this time, around 5–6 per cent of doctors and nurses were located in countries other than those of which they were nationals and they were concentrated in a handful of countries – Australia, Canada, West Germany, the UK and the USA (Mejia, Pizurki and Royston, 1979). In the decades since this study was published and especially since the 1990s, the scale of health professional migration has increased dramatically, migration flows have diversified beyond well know source countries such as India and the Philippines, and the belief that these movements are uncontrollable has been replaced with concerted efforts to manage migration within national and international arenas (OECD, 2007).

This chapter examines the causes and contours of health professional migration through the lens of one country's experience, the United Kingdom, focusing on the largest occupational group within health care, nurses, but also taking account of doctors' migration. Evidence from 17 European Countries and wider comparisons from beyond Europe indicated that the UK had the greatest reliance on foreign trained doctors of any OECD country (except New Zealand) and also made high usage of foreign trained nurses (Maier et al., 2011). Consistent with this picture, the UK, especially England, has been extremely active in the international migration of health professionals and also been prominent in seeking to manage migration via bilateral agreements between governments and the establishment of an ethical recruitment code of conduct. The chapter indicates that even in a context of increased global mobility and the free movement of labour within the European Union, governments retain scope to influence migration flows by adjusting immigration rules, altering licensing requirements and by signalling to employers, for example by establishing ethical recruitment codes, if international recruitment is to be utilised.

The Contribution of Migrant Health Professionals

Migrant health professionals have made an important contribution to the UK National Health Service (NHS) by boosting the size and diversity of the workforce, contributing to improvements in service delivery and by curtailing UK government expenditure on training. Concerns have been expressed by regulators and professional association about the quality and safety of care provided by some overseas trained health professionals, especially if education qualifications are not deemed to be genuinely equivalent or individuals lack adequate language competencies (British Medical Association, 2009; Nursing and Midwifery Council, 2005).

The reliance of the UK health system on overseas health workers has been influenced not only by distinctive features of the sector that provides greater scope for policy intervention but also the specific institutional context of the NHS. It forms part of central government and is financed from general taxation with the overwhelming majority of health services directly provided by the NHS with a relatively small, albeit growing, independent sector. The combination of state financing and provision has made the NHS susceptible to high levels of centralised control with major implications for staff, patients and the utilisation of overseas health professionals. Managerial and organisational reforms from the 1980s onwards strengthened accountability to the centre via elaborate systems of performance management ensuing overall workforce management remained firmly in the control of central government (Bach and Kessler, 2012). Workforce planning, however, has been erratic and workforce under-investment has been used to ensure tight control of staffing expenditure. This long-standing gap in domestic production of health professionals has been filled by reliance on non-EEA labour with a long history of employing overseas trained doctors and nurses (Raghuram and Kofman, 2002; Doyal, Hunter and Mellor, 1981).

The migration of health professionals has become a high profile and contentious political issue and this sensitivity has increased as more countries have been drawn into global migration flows. In addition there has been increased recognition of the centrality of adequate staffing levels and effective human resource management practice for health outcomes. This was symbolised, in 2006, by the World Health Organisation's focusing its annual flagship publication on issues of human resources for health, emphasising the centrality of the workforce for effective health outcomes. The WHO highlighted problems of staff shortages and noted that these challenges were exacerbated by international migration. Particular attention was focused on sub-Saharan Africa with the shortage of nurses and doctors hindering the achievement of the Millennium Development Goals (World Health Organisation, 2006). Affluent countries were criticised for undermining the capacity of countries to deliver adequate health care for its citizens. During the late 1990s the President of South Africa, Nelson Mandela, was highly critical of the active recruitment of South African nurses by the UK. This influenced the countries that the UK government considered it ethical to recruit from; sub-Saharan Africa was excluded as location for active recruitment.

Finally, the migration of health professionals is influenced strongly by the regulatory frameworks of individual governments that direct the training, recruitment and deployment of health professionals. One of the most prominent cases is the Philippines that has adopted a systematic policy of training nurses and other occupational groups for overseas employment. The state has put in place a series of policies to maximise the benefits of this loss of human capital via remittance income. The paradox is that at the same time as nurses leave the Philippines to work overseas, the government has insufficient resources to invest in its own health system to combat nurse shortages and poor working conditions (Ball, 2004).

Influences on Health Professional Migration

Migration has been analysed from a variety of disciplinary perspectives with limited consensus about its causes and consequences (Massey et al., 1998). A very widespread view is that migration is an inevitable component of globalisation and similar sentiments have been expressed in relation to the mobility of health professionals. According to Kingma (2007, p. 1,294), 'International mobility is a reality in a globalized world, one that will not be regulated out of existence'. As economic activity becomes more integrated and trade barriers decline so it is assumed that a global labour market is emerging in which all factors of production move around the world in search of the best returns. Globalisation may continue apace, although the global economic crisis has provided a salutary reminder that globalisation can be halted, as has occurred in previous eras. The emphasis on the *inevitability* of global mobility provides insufficient consideration of the extent to which other stakeholders, migrants themselves, employers and the nation state have an influence on the extent and types of mobility.

In contrast to the emphasis on structural factors associated with globalisation considerable attention has concentrated on the individual *agency* of the potential migrant; the emphasis is on the choices that individuals make. Neoclassical economic analysis suggests that migration flows stem from the existence of geographical wage differentials which are governed by the laws of supply and demand. Individuals compare the relative costs and benefits of remaining in their current country compared to the anticipated wage returns in moving to a new country. This theory's underlying approach is often abbreviated to focus on the push and pull factors that influence an individual's decision to migrate. Push factors encourage people to leave their country of origin and pull factors attract individuals to particular countries. Evidence from 17 EU countries suggests that income differentials were a key factor in many countries in encouraging exit. It was especially important amongst nurses and doctors in central and eastern countries, including Estonia, Poland and Romania, with opportunities to quadruple earnings in countries such as Germany. Poor working conditions were also frequently cited as a key driver of migration (Maier et al., 2011).

Wage differentials and unattractive working conditions are important components shaping migration, but as Massey et al. (1988) point out 'the existence of a wage differential still does not guarantee international movement, nor does its absence preclude it'. A limitation of the neoclassical approach is that by focusing solely on the aspirations of the individual migrant, a range of other actors, especially employers, that influence migrant behaviour are under-played (Bach, 2007; McGovern, 2007). Migration specialists have also noted the extent to which migration represents a household or community strategy to maximise income, with different roles allocated to household members. In the Philippines, women are often encouraged to become nurses because of the opportunities available to work abroad, spreading risk and bolstering household income (Ball, 2004).

As well as considering the motives of individuals and households, the supply side, the central role of employers in creating demand for migrant labour requires consideration. Piore (1979) suggested that migration stems from the structural demand for migrant labour within advanced industrial economies and it is only when employer demand stimulates migration that such flows occur. He argued that the use of migrant labour has specific advantages for employers that arise primarily from the attributes of jobs that migrants fill, rather than solely the wages that they are paid.

Migrants often fill jobs that are dirty, difficult, dangerous and demeaning. These jobs are not invariably low-paid but they usually denote low status with few opportunities for advancement. The labour market is segmented and native-born workers are disinclined to fill roles that are low status and stigmatised, as in the case of care work (Cangiano et al., 2009). In higher status professions like medicine there are certain less popular specialties (such as care of the elderly) or particular non-career grades that lie outside the main career structure that are hard to fill. Similarly, migrant health professionals have often been employed in under-served, usually remote, rural areas that have difficulties recruiting and retaining health workers.

Employers also draw on migrant labour because they are reluctant to raise wages to alleviate shortages that may have a knock on effect as higher paid workers seek to restore wage differentials. Moreover, migrant wage expectations are framed by the labour market in their country of origin, reducing their wage expectations, especially if they envisage a temporary stay abroad. Finally, Piore (1979) also noted that in addition to their influence on labour demand, employers also have a significant influence on immigration policy because they have a strong common interest in maintaining an open immigration regime and expend resources to lobby for such policies. By contrast opponents of immigration policy have diverse interests and may be influenced by immigration in diffuse and intangible ways, limiting effective opposition. Consequently some jobs that are unattractive to native-born workers are taken up by migrants, who are less influenced by social status and more concerned with immediate economic security. Employers exert influence over government to maintain an open migration regime. These influences are evident in the UK case.

UK Reliance on Overseas Health Professionals

There has been a long history of international recruitment in the NHS. In the 1950s successive Conservative governments adopted policies of cost containment which resulted in low pay and poor working conditions for nurses, exacerbating staff shortages (Carpenter, 1988). The government turned to its colonies and established the Colonial Nursing Service in 1940 to create an imperial labour market for nurses to assist in the recruitment of overseas nurses (Solano and Rafferty, 2007). In this period, shortages amongst doctors was also encouraging medical staff immigration, drawing on the UK's imperial legacy with India, the predominant source country (Kyriakides and Virdee, 2003). A period of heightened tension led to tighter immigration controls and the establishment of the work permit system in 1971. Provision was made, however, for overseas student nurses to undertake ward-based training and they were channelled into lower-tier enrolled nurse training and employed disproportionately in psychiatric and geriatric institutions. Mirroring current workforce patterns immigrant nurses and doctors have continued to be over represented in less popular specialties, grades and geographic locations (Oikelome and Healy, 2007).

Doyal's (1981) study published during the onset of recession also indicated how the state had responded to concerns that reductions in NHS expenditure could disadvantage home-based nurses. She reported that overseas nurses were having difficulty gaining a work permit because they were only being issued to newly-qualified overseas nurses if no home-based nurse could be recruited. Immigration controls were therefore being tightened up 'irrespective of the needs or desires of the [overseas] nurse themselves' (Doyal et al., 1981, p. 69). Similar state activism has been evident over the last decade with liberalisation followed by a tightening of immigration rules (Bach, 2010).

From the late 1990s the UK went through another period of active recruitment as more investment was channeled into the NHS and this resourcing was translated into workforce growth. There are a variety of data sources that can be used to assess these trends, but it is important to bear in mind that each source uses a different attribute of the migrant population. For example, Labour Force Survey (LFS) data examines occupational data by country of birth and nationality, but professional registration data focuses on the country that the individual obtained their professional qualification, that is, where they were trained. The main measure of the share of migrants in the workforce by nationality is the LFS. In 2002, health care professionals comprised 25 per cent of the workforce and this share increased to 29 per cent by 2008, following the wave of international recruitment. There was also a substantial increase in share amongst associate health professionals, with an increase from 14 to 18 per cent over the same time period (Aldin, James and Wadsworth, 2010). Further disaggregation indicates that amongst medical practitioners, in 2008, 32 per cent were born in non-EEA countries and five per cent were born in the EEA (excluding the UK). For nurses the respective figures were 19 and three per cent (cited in MAC, 2008, p. 288). Almost a third of medical practitioners and a fifth of nurses working in the UK health sector were therefore born outside the EEA and the relatively small proportion of EEA born nurses in the UK, indicated that the large influx of Central and East European workers after 2004 did not initially include a significant number of registered nurses.

More detailed data on stocks and flows can be gauged from the registration data provided by the General Medical Council (GMC) and the Nursing and Midwifery Council (NMC). To practice as a doctor or registered nurse in the UK, requires admission to the relevant professional register – GMC or NMC register. These registers provide data on the number of doctors, nurses and midwives on the register, information about where the individual qualified and the annual numbers entering and leaving the register, providing a good indication of workforce trends. The main drawback is that registration data only provides a proxy measure of employment because it registers intention to work rather than actual employment status.

Overall in 2012, 252,653 doctors were registered on the List of Registered Medical Practitioners (LRMP) (GMC, 2012). After the UK, India was the top country of qualification for doctors on the registrar, followed by Pakistan and South Africa (Table 9.1). Although there is considerable diversity of countries, the *stock* of doctors on the registrar highlights the legacy of doctors from the Indian sub-continent in the composition of the medical registrar, but the *flow* of new registrations provides an indication of how this has altered in recent years. GMC data indicates that typically over the last decade around 12,000 doctors (including full, temporary and provisional categories) join the register each year. There was a spike in new registrations amongst overseas trained doctors between 2003 and 2005; a very active period of overseas recruitment. A substantial proportion of these doctors were trained in Africa, India and Pakistan. For example, in 2003, there were 3,728 new registration by doctors trained in Africa, 174 per cent higher than in the previous year and in 2004 the number of registrations by doctors trained in India and Pakistan increased by 28 per cent and 96 per cent respectively compared to 2003. In the middle of the decade there was a surge in registrations from doctors trained in the EEA whilst non-EEA doctors started to reduce as restrictions were placed on non-EEA doctors (Blacklock et al., 2012).

For nurses, in 2012 670,000 midwives and health visitors were registered with the NMC. The number of new entrants to the register fluctuates considerably with UK registrations comprising around 15–20,000 per annum and this total has

Table 9.1   **Top 10 countries of qualification by primary medical qualification (PMQ), 8 November 2012**

PMQ country	Number of doctors	Per cent
United Kingdom	160,186	63.4
India	25,370	10.0
Pakistan	8,952	3.5
South Africa	5,724	2.3
Ireland	4,016	1.6
Nigeria	3,931	1.6
Germany	3,299	1.3
Egypt	3,129	1.2
Greece	2,635	1.0
Italy	2,469	1.0

Source: GMC, 2012.

usually exceeded international recruits (EU and non-EU). However, in 2001/02 this position was reversed for the first and only time as Figure 9.1 indicates.

Figure 9.1 indicates a sharp rise in registrations, especially from internationally trained nurses from the late 1990s until around 2004. There was then a sharp decline in new registrations until 2010 with the start of a modest recovery thereafter. In the period of sharpest decline after 2004, the number of new initial nurse registrations declined to 2,309 by 2008, a reduction of more than 80 per cent since 2004. Figure 9.1 also provides detail on the relative balance on inflows to the register from those trained in the UK compared to those from international sources (combining EU and non-EU sources). In the peak year of 2001/02, the number of non-EU nurse registrants exceeded those from the UK with only 47 per cent of new entrants qualified in the UK compared to almost 90 per cent in the early 1990s. By 2011/12, the composition of new entrants had returned to a position more akin to the position a decade earlier with UK qualified nurses providing the majority of new entrants, but in a context of a modest recovery international registrations.

Figure 9.2 indicates that registrations from EU countries (excluding the UK) have been more stable than non-EU countries because they are less subject to changes in immigration rules, but are influenced by other factors such as the impact of the economic crisis on job opportunities. Over the last decade as non-EU inflow was curtailed, EU registration did not initially increase substantially, but this pattern has altered in the last couple of years with EU countries representing the majority of the inflow. In terms of non-EU countries, the key source countries

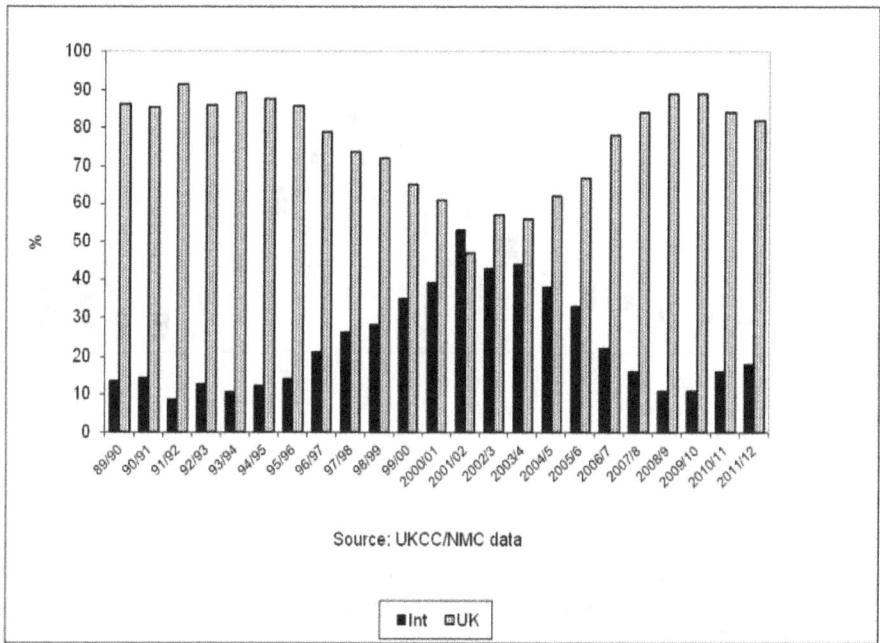

Source: UKCC/NMC data

■Int □UK

Figure 9.1   International and UK sources as a percentage of total new admissions to the UK nursing register, 1989/90 to 2011/12

Source: NMC/Buchan and Seccombe cited in RCN, 2012. Reproduced with kind permission of the Royal College of Nursing, from RCN Labour Market Review 2012, *Overstretched, Under-resourced.*

that contributed to the increase in the early part of the noughties were especially India, the Philippines and Australia. For example, in 1999 52 nurses from the Philippines registered, compared to 5,593 in 2003 (see Bach, 2007).

It is also worth noting that although this chapter concentrates on the active recruitment of overseas trained health professionals, the UK is also a very significant *source* country as well as a *destination* country for doctors and nurses. Nurses born in the UK comprise the second most important stock of immigrant nurses (after the Philippines) in the OECD. For doctors the UK is the third most important source country (after India and Germany). UK born doctors represent about 75 per cent of the immigrant doctors from the OECD in Ireland and New Zealand and more than 50 per cent in Australia (OECD, 2007, p. 173). These patterns account for some of the gap between registration data and employment data. Many UK-trained doctors and nurses maintain their UK registration and are included in the General Medical Council (GMC) and Nursing and Midwifery Council (NMC), although they are working outside the UK.

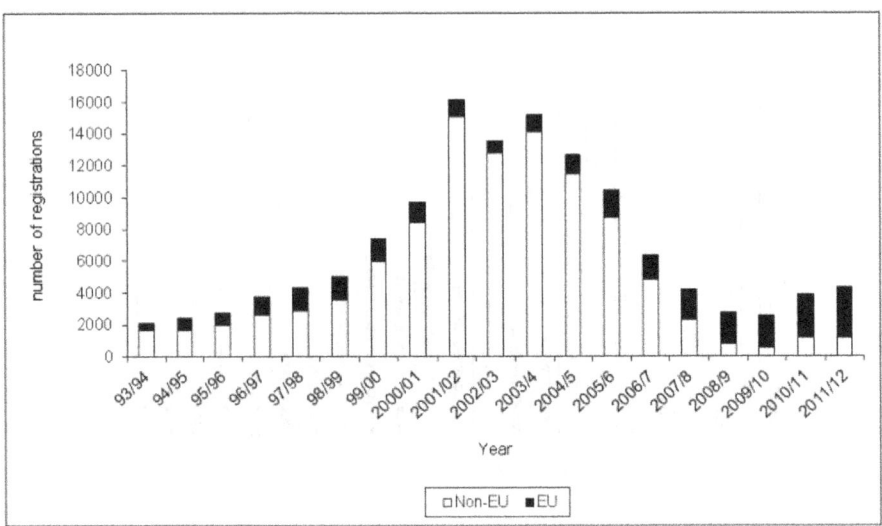

Figure 9.2   Admissions to the UK nursing register from EU countries and non-EU countries, 1993/94 to 2011/12

Source: NMC/Buchan and Seccombe cited in RCN, 2012. Reproduced with kind permission of the Royal College of Nursing, from RCN Labour Market Review 2012, *Overstretched, Under-resourced.*

Migration Governance: The Rise and Fall of International Recruitment

To make sense of these fluctuations in the international migration of health professionals it is instructive to divide the period since 1997 into three phases. Phase one was a period of active recruitment that covered the period between 1998 and 2005. Phase two, between 2006 and 2008, involved a recalibration of migration policy and a shifting perspective on the use of overseas health professionals. A more restrictive regime was instigated, but using the same institutional mechanisms as phase one, whilst phase three, from 2009, involved a major repositioning of immigration policy with the presumption of 'closure' except in exceptional circumstances. The NHS is especially sensitive to shifts in immigration policy because as a public sector employer, the government can exert direct control over NHS workforce policy. The extent of integration of NHS employer practice and state immigration policy highlights unambiguously the connections between state and employer policy in the use of migrant health professionals.

Phase one commenced after the Labour government took office in 1997 committed to addressing staff shortages, low morale and lengthy NHS waiting times. The scale of its ambition was revealed in the NHS Plan that unveiled unprecedented NHS investment and committed the NHS to employ 7,500 more consultants, 2,000 more GPs, 20,000 more nurses and 7,500 Allied Health

Professionals (therapists) by 2004 (Department of Health, 2000). These targets were exceeded and some targets were revised upwards, for example, for nurses the target was raised to 35,000 additional nurse posts by 2008. International recruitment was the preferred strategy to ensure rapid workforce growth because of the expense and lengthy lead times involved in increasing domestically trained nurses and doctors (Health Committee, 2007).

The Department of Health established an institutional infrastructure to facilitate recruitment activity. An NHS Director of International Recruitment was appointed, supported by International Recruitment Co-ordinators with the number of staff recruited internationally comprising a key performance target. These co-ordinators and staff located in embassies in Spain and elsewhere aided NHS trusts in their recruitment efforts. Financial support was made available, enabling managers to travel, to the Philippines in particular, to recruit batches of 50–100 nurses at a time. The Department of Health actively marketed the NHS through its website providing information about the cost of living and providing pen portraits of nurses who extolled the virtues of nursing in the UK. It also established a series of bilateral agreements with specific governments (India, Indonesia, Spain, Philippines, South Africa and China) that were willing to allow the UK to recruit because they had a surplus of a specific occupational group or viewed migration as an important source of remittance income. For medical staff, the NHS introduced a specific International Fellowship Programme in 2002 that offered substantial financial and practical support to facilitate mobility and the prospect of more permanent employment in the NHS if a suitable post became available.

Finally, the government eased immigration rules and the rigor with which those rules were implemented. For those outside the EEA, the work permit system had been the basis of the system with the granting of a work permit linked to employer sponsorship and skill level. The number of work permits was not subject to annual quotas but the Home Office published a National Shortage Occupation List which identified skill shortages. If jobs were not on the shortage list, in most circumstances employers had to undertake a resident labour market test, demonstrating that they had advertised their post for at least one week and provide reasons as to why they rejected applications from resident workers (Salt and Millar, 2006). This system provided a considerable degree of flexibility because the number of work permits allocated and the various channels used could all be adjusted facilitating relaxation or tightening of immigration rules without recourse to parliamentary approval.

At December 2004, almost 70 specialist health care occupations including consultant medical staff in a number of specialist areas, salaried GPs and dentists, nurses, midwives, dieticians, biomedical scientists, pharmacists, clinical psychologists, occupational therapists and language therapists were included in the Home Office health care shortage occupation list. This list signalled that the UK was seeking non-UK qualified health professionals. By comparison in June 2008, towards the end of the more restrictive phase two period, only medical consultants in a number of specific specialties were included in the shortage list as were very senior registered nurses, but not entry level registered nurses.

From 2006 until 2008 a more restrictive immigration policy was put in place with restrictions on accessing postgraduate training for doctors from outside the EEA and changes in the shortage occupational list for nurses and doctors. In July 2006, the government gave only six weeks' notice that it was removing general nurses (Band 5 and 6) from the government's shortage occupation list (Department of Health, 2006). Band 5 covers staff nurses, often newly qualified, to more experienced Band 6 nurses. This meant that an employer would have to demonstrate that they had advertised the vacancy and been unable to recruit a suitable UK or EEA applicant before applying to the Home Office for a work permit.

In what ways, did this shift in policy occur? The main impetus behind the international recruitment of nurses and other health professionals, staff targets, had been exceeded by 2005. The Health Committee (2007, p. 13) was critical of poor workforce planning and pointed out:

> The NHS Plan set a target for increasing nursing numbers by 20,000 between 1999 and 2004. In fact nursing numbers increased by more than 67,000 during this period, some 340 per cent in excess of the original target.

Around 2005/06, the NHS's and government's priorities started to shift from staff growth to curbing staff expenditure. This was against a backdrop of increased public concern about the far larger than anticipated influx of migrants from A8 [central and Eastern European] countries and emerging concerns about the sustainability of unprecedented increased NHS expenditure. The Labour government was also very sensitive to accusations that it was poaching nurses from less developed countries and exacerbating shortages of health professionals, leading it to adopt and subsequently revise an ethical recruitment code (Department of Health, 2001, 2004). The government also argued that international recruitment was only ever intended as a temporary measure whilst domestic nurse training provision was being increased. Between 1999 and 2005, the number of domestic nurse training places expanded rapidly from around 17,700 to 23,650 per annum, an increase of a third (Health Committee, 2007, p. 16). This expansion reflected a growing belief within the Department of Health that by 2006 'the NHS was largely self-sufficient' and any shortfall in nurse staffing could be addressed by 'health workers from East Europe' (Crisp, 2007, p. 120). This policy shift was reinforced by shifts in licensing requirements from 2005–2006 that made it more difficult for overseas nurses to gain NMC registration. Because of more onerous language and training requirements being put in place. As Figure 9.2 indicates, there was a sharp fall in non-EU registrations.

Phase three commenced at the end of 2008 and was the culmination of a shift from a relatively open, liberal immigration regime to a restrictive regime that actively discouraged the use of non-EEA health professionals. A key change was the introduction of the points based system (PBS) in 2008. The government used the discourse of global competition to argue that a new PBS would target skilled migrants that were essential to the UK's position in the world economy.

The system has been explicitly linked to economic requirements, with different degrees of eligibility to enter the UK based on a skill hierarchy with fewest restrictions on the most highly skilled. Underpinning the system, the government established an independent Migration Advisory Committee (MAC) to identify labour market shortages amongst skilled occupations and to recommend where it is sensible to fill that shortage via immigration from outside the EEA. The MAC recommended its first list of shortage occupations in September 2008 and this had the immediate effect of closing off most nursing jobs to non-EEA residents (see Bach, 2010). Since 2008, there have been continuous adjustments made to the PBS criteria, making them more demanding and thereby restricting the scope for non-EEA nurses and doctors to take up employment in the UK. These changes include raising the English language requirement threshold, increasing the minimum pay threshold and raising the skill level of the job (the skill level of the migrant is no longer assessed) to graduate level. In addition, the Coalition government is in the process of breaking the link between employment and residency. Previously, after five years migrants were granted permanent residency but the coalition government has ended this link and the likelihood is that it will lead to the removal of migrant nurses from the UK after they have worked in the UK for five years. The government's impact assessment suggests that '48% of migrant nurses would be excluded' (Boffey, 2012). In addition to qualitative criteria the coalition government has brought in quantitative criteria – an absolute cap on numbers.

These shifts in policy have also had consequences for the experience of being a migrant nurse. The experience of overseas nurses working in the UK has varied. Nurses often make use of recruitment agents that charge high fees to place nurses in employment and sometimes provide misleading information about the type of work and the geographical location of the workplace or promise jobs that do not materialise (Boseley, 2011). All nurses have to be registered with the UK professional nursing organisation before they can be employed as registered nurses and it can be difficult to gain the relevant placements and experience, resulting in qualified nurses working as health care assistants for much lower wages. In general nurses employed in the NHS and recruited in a systematic and structured way have a much more positive experience of employment with formal induction and mentoring (Young, 2011). This contrasts with nurses working in independent sector nursing homes that frequently confront issues of deskilling as their qualifications are not utilised and their experience discounted. Internationally recruited nurses want to be treated with respect by patients and other staff and not allocated poor shift patterns or provided with few training and promotion opportunities.

Conclusions

The health sector has a long history of employing migrant health professionals. It reflects the historical under-investment in the sector's workforce and scope in the past to encourage doctors and nurses, to come to the UK to complete their *training* and work in the NHS. These migrant workers gained access to training and ultimately gained citizenship, although at a cost in terms of being channelled into the least popular specialties and locations and experiencing widespread discrimination.

Since 1997, three distinct phases of state policy can be identified that has had a major impact on the receptiveness of the UK to overseas trained health professionals. After 1997, the Labour government actively sponsored a new phase of international recruitment. A combination of unprecedented increases in NHS expenditure, limited domestic supply and short-term targets to increase the NHS workforce led the government to encourage nurses and medical staff to come to the UK. The emphasis was on attracting *qualified* staff with less attention placed on training with a code of ethical recruitment and bilateral agreements developed, designed to forestall accusations of brain drain. By easing immigration rules, establishing an infrastructure to facilitate international recruitment – alongside the government's capacity to shape NHS employment policy – the outcome was a rapid expansion of migrant health professionals employed in the UK health system. The UK case therefore demonstrates the potential in a highly regulated and centralised health system for international recruitment to make an important contribution to achieving government workforce targets. In addition to the pivotal role of the UK government the increased importance of other institutions and actors are also evident, for example, the key role of the Philippines as a source country for the UK. This flow has been facilitated by the growth of recruitment agencies and by the deliberate state policy of encouraging emigration, in countries such as the Philippines (Masselink and Lee, 2010).

Since 2005, the public policy and labour market context has altered and the period of rapid expansion of the NHS workforce has ended. The UK has moved towards greater self-sufficiency in its health sector workforce and the shortages that existed in recent years have receded. This altered policy context has placed the burden of adjustment on migrant health professionals whose employment prospects have altered radically because of changes in UK immigration rules (Bach, 2010; RCN 2012). An especially contentious change was the removal of permit free training for International Medical Graduates (IMGs) who are not UK or EEA nationals. Until this change IMGs training or working in the UK did not require a work permit, but in Spring 2006 the government announced that permit free status would be rescinded within a month with detrimental consequences for IMG employment. In the aftermath of this controversy, attempts are being made to ensure that non-EEA doctors can undertake short-term clinical training in the UK under the auspices of the Medical Training Initiative. Similar concerns have been expressed by overseas nurses about unforeseen shifts in government policy with many non-EEA nurses facing the prospect of removal from the UK as successive government have continued to tighten and restrict criteria using the flexibility of the new Points Based System to bring about changes on an incremental basis with limited parliamentary scrutiny.

In tandem with most other OECD countries health expenditure as a proportion of GDP has increased over the last 50 years and the size of the workforce has expanded greatly. Underpinning the increase in migrant labour employed in the NHS since 1997 was unprecedented growth of the NHS budget. This period has ended and workforce investment has been arrested by the advent of the economic crisis with major consequences for the health care workforce. Although employment opportunities in the NHS have been reduced, this may not discourage international migration from within the European Union as employment and working conditions have deteriorated in many Central and Eastern European countries that may encourage further exit. The Coalition government is completing the shift from workforce investment to downsizing and austerity with reduced commissioning of nurse training. Consequently as the economy recovers it can be anticipated that shortages will re-emerge and the claims of 'self-sufficiency' will look increasingly hollow and another cycle of boom and bust will be initiated.

References

Aldin, V., James, D. and Wadsworth, J., 2010. The Changing Shares of Migrant Labour in Different Sectors and Occupations in the UK Economy: An overview. In: M. Ruhs and B. Anderson, eds. 2010. *Who Needs Migrant Workers? Labour shortages, immigration and public policy*. Oxford: Oxford University Press. pp. 57–85.

Bach, S., 2007. Going Global? The regulation of nurse migration in the UK. *British Journal of Industrial Relations*, 45(2), pp. 383–404.

———, 2010. Managed Migration? Nurse recruitment and the consequences of state policy. *Industrial Relations Journal*, 41(3), pp. 249–66.

Bach, S. and Kessler, I., 2012. *The Modernisation of the Public Services and Employee Relations: Targeted change*. London: Palgrave Macmillan.

Baldock, C., Heneghan, C., Mant, D. and Ward A., 2012. Effect of UK Policy on Medical Migration: A time series analysis of physician registration data. *Human Resources for Health*, 10(1), p. 35.

Ball, R., 2004. Divergent Development, Racialised Rights: Globalised labour markets and the trade of nurses – the case of the Philippines. *Women's Studies International Forum*, 27(2), pp. 119–33.

Boffey, D., 2012. Patient Care 'Will Suffer' Under Plans to Throw Out Migrant Nurses. *The Observer*, 25 March. [online] Available at: <http://www.theguardian.com/uk/2012/mar/25/migrant-nurses-nhs> [Accessed 19 December 2013].

Boseley, S., 2011. Nursing Dreams Turn Sour as Jobs in UK Disappear. *The Guardian*, 23 February.

British Medical Association, 2009. *BMA Response to the European Commission Green Paper on the European Workforce for Health*. London: British Medical Association.

Cangiano, A., Shutes, I., Spencer, S. and Leeson, G., 2009. *Migrant care workers in ageing societies: Research findings in the United Kingdom.* Oxford: Compas.

Carpenter, M., 1988. *Working for Health: The history of COHSE.* London: Lawrence and Wishart.

Castles, S., 2004. Why Migration Policies Fail. *Journal of Ethnic and Racial Studies,* 27(2), pp. 205–27.

Crisp, N., 2007. *Global Health Partnerships: The UK contribution to health in developing countries.* London: Department of Health.

Department of Health, 2000. *NHS Plan.* London: Department of Health.

———, 2001. *Code of Practice for NHS Employers.* London: Department of Health.

———, 2004. *Code of Practice for the International Recruitment of Healthcare Professionals.* London: Department of Health.

———, 2006. *Supporting UK nurses – Band 5 nurses to be taken off the Home Office shortage occupation list.* DH Press Release (2006/0256), 3 July.

Doyal, L., Hunt, G. and Mellor, J., 1981. Your Life in Their Hands: Migrant workers in the National Health Service. *Critical Social Policy,* 1(2), pp. 54–71.

GMC, 2012. *List of Registered Medical Practitioners – Statistics.* London: GMC.

Health Committee, 2007. *Workforce Planning: Fourth chapter of session 2006–07.* Volume 1 (HC-171-1). London: HMSO.

Hollifield, J., 2008. The Politics of International Migration: How can we 'bring the state back'? In: C. Brettel and J. Hollifield, eds. 2008. *Migration Theory, Talking Across Disciplines.* Second edition. London: Routledge, pp. 183–239.

Kingma, M., 2007. Nurses On the Move: A global overview. *Health Services Research,* 42(3), pp. 1,281–98.

Kyriakides, C. and Virdee, S., 2003. Migrant Labour, Racism and the British National Health Service. *Ethnicity and Health,* 8(4), pp. 283–305.

Maier, C., Glinos, I., Wismar, M., Bremner, J., Dussault, G. et al., 2011. Cross-Country Analysis of Health Professional Mobility in Europe: The results. In: M. Wismar, C. Maier, I. Glinos, G. Dussault and J. Figueras, eds. 2011. *Health Professional Mobility and Health Systems: Evidence from 17 European countries.* Copenhagen: European Observatory of Health Systems and Policies, ch. 2.

Masselink, L. and Lee, D., 2010. Nurses Inc.: Expansion and commercialization of nursing education in the Philippines. *Social Science and Medicine,* 71(1), pp. 166–72.

Massey, D., Arango, J., Hugo, G., Kouaouchi, A., Pellegrino, A. et al., 1998. *Worlds in Motion.* Oxford: Oxford University Press.

McGovern, P., 2007. Immigration, Labour Markets and Employment: Problems and prospects. *British Journal of Industrial Relations,* 45(2), pp. 217–35.

Mejia, A., 1978. Migration of Physicians and Nurses: A world wide picture. *International Journal of Epidemiology,* 7(3), pp. 207–15.

Mejia, A., Pizurki, H. and Royston, E., 1979. *Physician and Nurse Migration: Analysis and policy implications.* Geneva: WHO.

Migration Advisory Committee, 2008. *Skilled, Sensible, Shortage: The recommended shortage occupation lists for the UK and Scotland*. London: Migration Advisory Committee.

Nursing and Midwifery Council, 2005. *EU Language Position a 'Dangerous Farce' Says NMC President*. Press release, 44/2005.

OECD, 2007. Immigrant Health Workers in OECD Countries in the Broader Context of Highly Skilled Migration. *International Migration Outlook – Sopemi 2007 Edition*. Paris: OECD.

———, 2012. *Health at a Glance*. Paris: OECD.

Oikelome, F. and Healy, G., 2007. Second CLASS doctors? The impact of a professional career structure on the employment conditions of overseas and UK Qualified Doctors. *Human Resource Management Journal*, 17(2), pp. 134–54.

Piore, M., 1979. *Birds of Passage*. Cambridge: Cambridge University Press.

Raghuram, P. and Kofman, E., 2002. The State, Skilled Labour Markets, and Immigration: The case of doctors in England. *Environment and Planning A*, 34(11), pp. 2,071–89.

RCN, 2012. *Overstretched, Under-Resourced. The UK nursing labour market review 2012*. London: RCN.

Salt, J. and Millar, J., 2006. International Migration in Interesting Times: The case of the UK. *People and Place*, 14(2), pp. 14–24.

Solano, D. and Rafferty, A., 2007. Can Lessons be Learned from History? The origins of the British imperial nurse labour market. *International Journal of Nursing Studies*, 44(6), pp. 1,055–63.

Young, R., 2011. A Major Destination Country: The United Kingdom and its changing recruitment policies. In: M. Wismar, C. Maier, I. Glinos, G. Dussault and J. Figueras, eds. 2011. *Health professional mobility and health systems: Evidence from 17 European countries*. Copenhagen: European Observatory of Health Systems and Policies, ch.11.

World Health Organisation, 2006. *World Health Report 2006 – Working together for health*. Geneva: WHO.

PART IV
Regulating Bodies Across Borders

Chapter 10

Medical Tourism for Services Legal in the Home and Destination Country: Legal and Ethical Issues

Glenn Cohen

Introduction

'Medical tourism' (to use the most common term, though 'cross-border health care' or 'medical travel' could also be used), is the travel of patients from their home country to a foreign country for the primary purpose of receiving health care services. There is no doubt that the existing market is significant, even though there are considerable disputes about its exact size (Cohen, 2013; Cortez, 2011, p. 878). One set of estimates suggested roughly 750,000 US patients travelled abroad in 2007 for medical procedures (Cortez, 2011, p. 878; Murphy, 2009; Ehrbeck, Guevar and Mango, 2008, pp. 2–6). In 2004, more than 150,000 foreigners sought medical treatment in India, and that number was projected to increase by 15 per cent per year (Lancaster, 2004). In 2005, Bumrungrad International Hospital in Bangkok saw 400,000 foreign patients (Milstein and Smith, 2006, p. 1,638). In one year alone, it was estimated that 952,000 California residents traveled to Mexico for medical care or prescription drugs (Wallace, Mendez-Luck and Castañeda, 2009, p. 662). The revenues involved in this trade are also very impressive, with some claiming that medical tourism in India generated \$2.2 billion in revenues by 2012, and that it will generate \$8 billion in Thailand between 2010 and 2014 (Cohen, 2010, p. 1,472). If insurer-prompted medical tourism picks up in the US, as myself and other scholars expect, the volume and revenue flow is likely to expand even further; indeed, already each of the four largest insurer plans in the US have introduced or are considering introducing plans involving medical tourism (Cohen, 2010b, pp. 1,486–8; Cortez, 2011 pp. 882–4). The European market for medical tourism is poised to continue growing as well, especially now that there is a new European Union Directive on the subject that I will discuss below (Cohen, 2014; European Parliament, 2011).

These numbers are only a part of the story. To better understand the legal and ethical issues posed by medical tourism, I find it useful to categorise medical tourism in two separate ways (Cohen, 2012a). The first division is by patient population, of which there are three broad categories. First, there are patients paying out-of-pocket. In the US, this population includes uninsured or underinsured patients using medical tourism to achieve substantial cost savings and those seeking to use services unavailable at home; in universal health care systems, this group also includes patients seeking to queue jump (Cohen, 2010b). A second group consists of patients engaged in private insurer-prompted medical tourism. In its weakest form, insurers simply cover the service abroad without any incentive, but in a more common form, 'tourism-incentivized plans', individuals are offered rebates, waived deductibles or other payment incentives for receiving treatment abroad (Cohen, 2010b; Einhorn, 2008). A final group consists of patients engaged in government-prompted or covered medical tourism. For example, there have been recent proposals to give US Medicare and Medicaid patients incentives to use medical tourism another version is already in place in the EU, a matter I discuss below (Cohen, 2010b, 2014; Baker and Rho, 2009).

This chapter concerns legal and ethical issues related only to medical tourism for services that are *legal* in the patient's home and destination country and will cover issues faced by all three populations of medical tourists engaged in it: patients paying out of pocket, private insurer prompted and government prompted medical tourists. I put to one side medical tourism for services *illegal* in the home or destination country, which I have dealt with elsewhere (Cohen, 2010a, 2014). First, I will discuss the question of how tourist patients can determine the quality of foreign facilities, the possibility of state interventions and the ability and the provision of patient safety information and the challenges in securing that information are discussed, including comparisons to domestic initiatives. Second, and especially as to medical tourists coming from the US, I discuss the question of whether medical tourists can recover for medical malpractice committed abroad and possible regulatory salves. Third, I turn to private insurer prompted medical tourism, focusing on its existing (and potential) regulation in the US health care system. Finally, I discuss government-prompted medical tourism in the form of the EU rules regarding reimbursement of cross-border health care. Because of the large numbers of topics covered here, my treatment of each will be brief, but I have written on each in-depth in other work (Cohen, 2010a; 2010b; 2014).

Information on Foreign Facilities and Their Quality

Suppose an uninsured patient from the US is considering whether to go to India for a hip replacement, which she/he would pay for out of pocket. Part of what makes the Indian hospital attractive is that it will perform the procedure at one fifth the price she/he would pay in the US, which will result in significant savings to the patient even once travel costs and time off work are factored in (Cohen, 2010b). Indeed, as will often be the case with US uninsured patients seeking non-emergency care through medical tourism, the patient would not be able to afford the procedure in the US at its US price.

One major question our hypothetical patient will want to know is the quality of the care available at the Indian hospital. It turns out that this piece of information will be quite hard to acquire. Foreign countries by and large 'do not require their hospitals to measure and report surgical outcomes or to participate in international-performance measurement systems' (Cohen, 2010b; Milstein and Smith, 2006, p. 1,639). While, as World Bank economists Mattoo and Rathindran observe in an article in *Health Affairs*, it is certainly true that 'on average' the 'quality of care available in developing countries is lower than in industrialized countries', the 'relevant comparison is not with the standard of an average developing-country provider but with the standard of a provider likely to be used by [the medical-tourist patient] in their home country', (Mattoo and Rathindran, 2006, p. 359) and how they compare to the kind of care a particular patient could get domestically. For many uninsured or underinsured home country patients, the counterfactual is no non-emergency care at all.

Still, whatever evaluative baseline one adopts against which to evaluate the quality of foreign hospitals, one still needs to assess their quality. That information is very hard to get. A few small-scale empirical studies of specific therapies and hospitals suggest high quality care. Arnold Milstein and Mark Smith (2006, p. 1637 'doubt' that the average US hospital can 'offer better outcomes for common complex operations such as coronary-artery bypass grafting, for which several JCI-accredited offshore hospitals report gross mortality rates of less than 1%'. Mattoo and Rathindran (2006, p. 359) single out Bumrungrand Hospital in Bangkok, Apollo Hospital in New Delhi and Crossroads Center in Antigua as 'examples of reputable medical facilities in developing countries that are comparable to the best in industrial countries' and note that the Apollo hospital chain has maintained a 99 per cent success rate in more than 50,000 cardiac surgeries performed, which is 'on par with surgical success rates of the best US cardiac surgery centers'. However, Leigh Turner (2013) has recently compiled a list of several reports of death or serious injury connected to poor quality of care at destination hospitals, and it is hard to know if there are many more than have not been publicly discussed due to settlement agreements with confidentiality clauses or the difficulties in bringing suit I will discuss below.

A different way of trying to determine quality of foreign hospitals might be to look at indicia of quality touted by foreign hospitals, of which there are three primary ones: First, many hospitals champion the fact that they are Joint Commission International (JCI) accredited. JCI is an affiliate of the Joint Commission (formerly called the Joint Commission on Accreditation of Healthcare Organizations (JCAHO)), which accredits most US hospitals for participation in the Medicare and Medicaid programmes through a similar process. As I described the JCI requirements in 2010:

> To qualify for JCI hospital accreditation, the hospital must achieve the requisite scores on JCI's six patient goals and its more than 100 standards, which are divided into ten chapters. Each hospital is fully evaluated at the time of initial accreditation and at the time of reaccreditation every three years. When an evaluation shows that one or more conditions for accreditation are not met, the organization is provided a period of time to come into acceptable compliance

demonstrated by written proof or by a follow-up visit by one of the JCI evaluators. (Cohen, 2010b, p. 1,485)

Second, many foreign hospitals spotlight the extent to which their staff are made up of foreign-trained health care providers that have been deemed qualified to practice in the United States. Third, some foreign hospitals point to collaborations they have with US medical centres, such as partners Harvard Medical International, the Cleveland Clinic, and John Hopkins International (Cohen, 2010b, pp. 1,484–5).

While a patient may learn something from the fact that a foreign facility is JCI accredited, staffed by US trained providers or affiliated with a US hospital, these indicia alone are far from sufficient in determining whether the foreign facility is of high quality, and indeed we have no strong evidence that these indicia relate to the kinds of measures of quality that patients and policy-makers care about: mortality, morbidity, rate of hospital-acquired infections, avoidable injuries etc.. While some of the industry leaders like Bumungrad and Apollo have been studied as to some of these dimensions as to some forms of treatment (cardiac care has received the most quality assessments), foreign hospitals are radically different from one another and the quality of care they offer is likely to be very heterogeneous, with few reliable ways of telling them apart.

At the same time, it is important to recognise that this statement is also very much true of the US health care market. The US patient seeking health care within the United States faces well-documented disparities in hospital-care quality depending on location (Chandra and Skinner, 2004, p. 604). Further, a US patient trying to select the best hospital for a procedure is also plagued with deep and difficult-to-correct informational deficits as well as bounded-rationality problems in using that information. That is, '[p]atients often cannot assess the quality of care they receive, either before or after it is delivered' and, though in 'theory, patients can attempt to correct their information deficiencies by acquiring the necessary information', doing so is very costly as is using the information (Madison, 2007, pp. 1,583–4).

The question is what can we do to improve patient access to quality information as to medical tourism? Home country governments lack the direct power to force foreign hospitals to disclose information. Foreign hospitals and governments seeking to promote their medical tourism business may have an incentive to voluntarily disclose such information so as to signal their quality to consumers. But these reports may be prone to selective reporting, puffery or even fraud (Cohen, 2010b, p. 1,508).

What we really need is for JCI (or another third party institution if JCI is seen as too 'in the pocket' of foreign hospitals) to audit these error rates or publish them itself as a condition of accreditation. Alternatively, the US or another government or intergovernmental bodies could itself maintain the list and report the outcomes the way the US Centers for Disease Control and Prevention (CDC) does for fertility clinic success rates (42 USC. §263a-5(1)(A)), audit it periodically and exclude those whose data proved false. Elsewhere I have argued for this among other interventions that I call 'channelling', where home countries create conditions for foreign providers to get on an 'approved' list (such as disclosing certain mortality and morbidity information, or maintaining acceptable audited rates as to those things) wherein insurers, home country governments and patients are given incentives to use these facilities rather than 'unapproved' providers, as a way of trying to improve information disclosure and quality (Cohen, 2010b).

Even if we achieved sufficient information disclosure by foreign providers, there is the further question as to what that information could be compared to. While some US states such as New York and Pennsylvania have produced 'report cards' on facilities, they have used widely different measures, making comparisons between providers in different states quite difficult, let alone comparisons between providers in a particular US state and those abroad (Cohen, 2010b, pp. 1,507–8). But even if we achieved good disclosure of high quality information about hospitals in the patient's home and destination countries transformed that information into a standard set of metrics, the domestic experience with these kinds of informational interventions should lead us to measured expectations of how meaningfully they will improve patient choice. For report-card systems like the one in place in the US states of Pennsylvania and New York for cardiac care, there are ongoing debates about whether these devices contain accurate measures or whether patient-selection problems and cream skimming to 'game' the system skew the data (Cutler et al., 2004, p. 345). Even if we were convinced that the information contained in these reports was good, prior work suggests that patients fail to make use of that information because of bounded-rationality problems. Carl Schneider and Mark Hall, for example, have collected decades of empirical work on these problems to show doctors' reluctance to help patients make choices as health care consumers, patients' failure to understand health care delivery and statistics, patients' tendency to avoid making medical decisions and patients' fixation on cost over quality (Schneider and Hall, 2009). A Kaiser Family Foundation survey from 2000 surveyed 2,014 adult Americans and found that only roughly 10 per cent of Americans had used information comparing quality among health plans, hospitals and doctors, when available, that respondents favoured recommendations from friends, family and other doctors over actual data on health care quality in making provider selections, and that empirical studies of the New York and Pennsylvania report-card systems suggest the same (Cohen, 2010b; The Kaiser Family Foundation, 2000; Frank, 2004, pp. 20–21).

How well these bounded-rationality problems translate to medical tourism remains to be seen. While over-optimism, bias and trust in their US physicians cause many American patients to fail to use quality information about domestic providers, things may be different for medical tourism; it is possible that Americans may have inaccurately negative views of foreign physicians, in part because of an availability heuristic fuelled by negative depictions of unsanitary, third-world hospitals from film and television. Second, those paying for medical tourism out-of-pocket are already sick and may be more likely to consult report cards than the average American respondent that is the focus of the aforementioned domestic studies. Third, given the current minimal penetration of the medical-tourism industry in the US market, at present these patients are unlikely to have friends, family or primary-care providers to advise them on providers abroad once they have decided to use medical tourism. They may pay more attention to objective information than do their counterparts seeking domestic care who instead attach a lot of weight to recommendations from those they know. If the industry expands, though, this point of distinction from the domestic context is likely to diminish, and it may be less true for certain pockets of the existing market – for example, Californians of Mexican descent who go to Mexico for medical tourist services may already have such informal informational sources.

Still, my own reading of the existing literature leads me to doubt that mere information disclosure is enough. Instead I have argued in-depth elsewhere that we should adopt a more muscular form of the 'channeling' approach, whereby to be 'approved' (and thus be eligible for private or public insurer prompted medical tourists, or patients seeking to use tax deductions of cost, etc.) we require not the mere disclosure of information or something like the procedural-based JCI accreditation, but instead require that actual morbidity, mortality, avoidable error and hospital-acquired infection rates be below a level set by regulators. While individual patients paying out of pocket would still be free to go to 'unapproved' centres that do not meet these standards, by directing the funding of insured patients and by trying to steer patients paying out-of-pocket to approved centres, the hope is to create a strong incentive for foreign facilities to meet the approval criteria and improve quality for all their patients (for more in-depth discussion see Cohen, 2010b).

Medical Malpractice Recovery

Apart from concerns about quality of care is the question of recovery when medical tourism leads to medical errors. To be sure, the two issues are not entirely separate to the extent liability rules deter medical error, something that is contested in the domestic medical malpractice literature (Frakes, 2012; Currie and MacLeod, 2008; Greenberg et al., 2010).

US medical tourists (as well as those from many other home countries) will face a series of difficulties in recovering for medical error that occurred abroad: difficulties in establishing personal jurisdiction over the defendants, in avoiding dismissal on the ground of *forum non conveniens*, in enforcing judgments patients do achieve and in getting around the fact that much less remunerative foreign laws will often apply to an action even if it can be brought in a US court. If patients are unable to bring suit and must sue in the destination country to recover, the delays and expenses are very discouraging and likely to render a lawsuit non-viable (Cohen, 2010b; Cortez, 2010, p. 10).

Facilitators who recruit patients in the patient's home country are more likely to be amenable to suit there. The same is true of insurers, who are ordinarily based in the home country and clearly subject to its jurisdiction. However, at least in the

US, the available legal theories for recovery against these entities are much less plaintiff-friendly than those available against foreign providers, such that patients are less likely to be able to successfully sue (Cohen, 2010b; 2014).

The question is what to make of this gap between patients treated in the home country and those treated through medical tourism? In the US, and in many home countries, we prohibit individuals from contracting with their domestic physician to waive medical malpractice recovery in exchange for a better price. Medical tourism allows patients to circumvent this prohibition. That might seem problematic, but as I have argued elsewhere a number of additional factors serve to mitigate this problem: it has to be considered against the backdrop of the permissibility of *intra*national medical tourism and its medical malpractice effects, the toleration of agreements to arbitrate malpractice disputes, the ability of patients to self-insure against potential recovery difficulties through specialised insurance products and certain key legal and economic differences between contracting for less compensatory legal rules and travelling to locations that have such rules (Cohen, 2010b).

If worried about the lack of recovery, a home country could attempt more muscular 'channelling' regimes that required foreign facilities to, for instance, engage in agreements to arbitrate, consent to jurisdiction or offer medical malpractice insurance as a condition of accreditation by third-party accreditors like JCI, or to be on the 'approved' list of national or international regulators. As I will discuss in a moment, for private insurer-prompted medical tourism such measures are even easier to implement and the US state of California has adopted a somewhat analogous system in licensing insurance products covering travel to Mexico for care (Cohen, 2010b).

More radically, home countries could attempt to create victim's compensation funds (in analogy to the September 11th Victim's Compensation Fund or the Worker's Compensation system in the US, to compensate medical tourists for injuries abroad (Cohen, 2012a, 2014; Sawicki, 2012, p. 653). Such a scheme could be funded by levying a fee on facilities that wished to be part of the 'approved' list in the 'channelling' regime and using that revenue to pay for this system, or by charging facilitators who recruit in the US. Alternatively, funding could come from charging insurers using medical tourism (discussed below) a per-patient fee and using that revenue to cross-subsidise the no-fault compensation system for uninsured patients (Cohen, 2012a, 2014. It could also create regimes of expanded vicarious liability for facilitators and insurers (Cohen, 2010b, 2014).

Private Insurer-Prompted Medical Tourism

As Nathan Cortez and I have reported in our prior work, private insurers in the US are beginning to incorporate medical tourism in their plans. The four largest commercial insurers in the United States (UnitedHealth, WellPoint, Aetna, and Humana) have either introduced medical tourism pilot programmes or are considering it; BlueCross BlueShield of South Carolina contracted with a hospital in Bangkok, Thailand, to perform certain surgeries; 200 US employers offer a network of foreign providers through BasicPlus Health Insurance, which sells group plans and contracts with medical tourism facilitator Companion Global Healthcare. As of 2006, United Group Programs, a third-party insurance administrator, had contracted to outsource surgeries for at least forty US companies. And Blue Ridge Paper Products in North Carolina and the Hannford Brothers Supermarket in New England made headlines when they announced plans to send employees abroad. In California, a state which has been the most far-reaching in its attempt to regulate private insurer prompted medical tourism, Health Net, Blue Shield, and Mexican insurer SIMNSA offer plans to California residents willing to be treated in Mexico, at prices costing 40–50 per cent less than those that confine insurance to those domestically (Cohen, 2010b; Cortez, 2011, pp. 882–4).

We are only at the tip of the iceberg here. What might these new plans look like? As against the status quo (call it 'SQ') private insurance plans covering health care only in the home country, we might imagine medical tourism being incorporated in four ways. Tourism Covered ('TC') plans would cover health care sought in approved facilities abroad without giving additional incentives to use it as against the SQ plan, instead it would give patients the *option* to use medical tourism with no inducement to do so. Tourism Incentivized ('TI') plans would cover care at home the same way SQ does, but provide patients an incentive to use medical tourism for certain procedures at certain foreign hospitals by the waiver of a deductible or sharing some of the cost savings with patients or other incentives. The State of West Virginia debated legislation that would have introduced this kind of plan for its public employees, and Hannford Supermarkets (a large employer in the American northeast) was poised to introduce such a plan (Cohen, 2010b; Einhorn, 2008; H.B. 4359, 77th Leg., 2d Sess. (W. Va. 2006)). Domestic Extra ('DE') plans would cover US-based treatment for all medical procedures the same way as Plan SQ, except, the patient would pay extra for a schedule procedure if they elected to have that procedure performed by a US doctor, for example through a higher co-pay. Finally, Tourism Mandatory ('TM') plans would be similar to DE plans, but differ in that the insurer will not cover the specified non-emergency procedure *at all* if the procedure is performed domestically. The patient may still elect to seek the procedure domestically rather than at Apollo, but must pay out of pocket (Cohen, 2010b, pp. 1,447–8, 1,556).

This is a very skeletal articulation of the potential market, and there is in fact an extremely large number of possible plans that will differ (for starters) on four dimensions: 1) Does the insurer use positive incentives (for example, premium rebates for selecting foreign care) or negative incentives (for example, higher co-pays for domestic care) to induce medical tourism or simply refuse to cover treatment domestically, and what are the sizes of the incentives if used? 2) For what services? 3) At which foreign hospitals? 4) If a procedure is covered in more than one foreign hospital, is the patient given a choice among them? Plans can get much more complicated: refusing to cover domestic care at all for some services while requiring a co-pay for others, setting differential pricing of the co-pays as between different foreign hospitals from which the patient can choose etc. (Cohen, 2010b).

The same quality and med-mal recovery issues that plague medical tourism by patients paying out-of-pocket are also present here. Indeed, there may be more reason to be concerned, in that patients are making a precommitment at the time of enrolment rather than at the point of service and may face choice paralysis, information overload and other bounded rationality problems in choosing between potential plans (Cohen, 2010b). On the other hand as I have argued in-depth elsewhere, insurers have a greater capacity and incentive to evaluate the quality of the providers to which they send patients and to select higher quality providers. The patient and the insurers' incentive is, to be sure, not perfectly aligned because US patients switch insurers relatively frequently. Recent empirical work suggests that 16.6 per cent of privately insured adults changed their insurer within a 12-month period, most frequently (38.5 per cent of the time) due to a change in the insured's own or spouse's employer (Cohen, 2010b; Herring, 2010) – such that insurers do not fully internalise the benefits or burdens that providers of various quality place on their patients. Nevertheless, because US insurers can save considerable costs and improve profit margins by getting insured patients to use medical tourism, they have some incentive to select high-quality foreign providers in order to achieve good reputational effects and foster the development of a robust private insurer medical tourism market.

Moreover, since for many forms of health insurance in the US states retain large amounts of regulatory authority, regulation could fairly easily be implemented to better align the interests of insurers and patients through a number of 'channelling' interventions. As I have discussed in much greater depth elsewhere (Cohen, 2010b), we could allow insurer-prompted medical tourism only for a list of approved services that we think pose the smallest risk to the patient, or based on whether the facility has done a fixed number of a particular service in the last calendar year. We could prohibit insurers from incentivising or requiring tourism with providers unless they are JCI-accredited, meet a threshold requirement of US trained or certified doctors, or are partnered with high-quality US institutions. Again, states could go further and construct their own 'approval' criteria based on required disclosures with periodic auditing and review, although that would introduce greater costs and complexity. An intermediate approach might be based on some Preferred Provider Organisation (PPO) statutes that require quality-management programmes, sometimes requiring that a physician lead them. We could also require insurers to cover domestically all follow-up care from surgeries provided abroad as an attempt to try and mitigate some of the concerns that have been raised about continuity of care.

Similarly, we could institute measures aimed at dampening the med-mal-recovery-disparity problems by prohibiting insurers from using providers who did not enter consent-to-jurisdiction agreements (or otherwise subject themselves to jurisdiction in the state), forum-selection agreements, choice-of-law agreements and/or maintain assets in the state. A different way of achieving some of this benefit would be to require insurers to contract with a third-party insurer for medical-tourist medical-malpractice insurance of the kind discussed above. Instead of seeking compensation for the medical error from the foreign provider, the patient would now be able to achieve compensation from this third-party. Each of these interventions could be applied for some types of plans but not others (for example, TM and DE but not TI).

A separate set of reforms worth thinking about is the regulation of the various plan designs that are made available in the market. The most modest intervention for employer-sponsored health insurance, which is also libertarian paternalist, would be to use the stickiness of defaults in favour of SQ plans by requiring that, when offering patients the choice, the SQ plan is treated as the default option. The most muscular intervention would be to outlaw certain plan types altogether, for example prohibit TM or DE plans from being offered, which is one way of reading what the US state of Texas has attempted to do (Cohen, 2010b; Tex. Ins. Code Ann. §121.004 (Vernon, 2009)). An intermediate approach would take inspiration from existing regulation of PPO and Health Maintenance Organisation (HMO) plans in the domestic US health care market. This would lead us, among other things, to directly regulate the co-pays insurers are allowed to charge for each procedure in both its domestic and medical-tourism variety. More administrable variants could either be modelled on some PPO statutes that establish maximum fixed disparities in co-pays (20–25 per cent in some PPO statutes), require that the disparity be cost justified, or a hybrid one that sets a presumption that no co-pay or rebate disparity will exceed a set per cent but allows the insurer to justify greater disparities on the ground that they are cost justified (Cohen, 2010b).

Importantly, because of the pre-emption effect of the Employee Retirement Income Security Act ('ERISA') statute, most state insurance law will *not* govern self-insured firms, which is a nontrivial problem since self-insured firms are a large part of the US Market (Cohen, 2010b; 29 USC. §1144(b) (2)(B) (2006)). While it is possible that regulations aimed at regular private insurers will influence medical tourism providers, producing spill over benefits for self-insured firms, a much more direct and assured solution would be for the US federal government to legislate directly.

Medical Tourism and Public Health Insurance: The EU Model

In the US the major legal issues have surrounded quality, medical malpractice recovery and the regulation of private insurance products, discussed above. In Europe the conversation has been quite different and has revolved around medical tourism by patients from one EU member state (the 'Member State of Affiliation') to another (the 'Member State of Treatment') and rules about authorisation and payment.

The EU has no single health care system. Instead the member states that make up the EU retain competency in this area and each provides health care to its nationals. In part due to differences between EU health care systems, medical tourism remains popular within the EU and providers can and do offer a vastly different array of services and technologies from one member state to another, much more so than between US states (Cohen, 2014; Flear, 2007).

The central aim of the European Union project was and continues to be economic integration, achieved primarily through the breaking down of barriers, hindrances or restrictions to the four fundamental freedoms of the EU internal market – goods, services, persons and capital (Consolidated Version of the Treaty on European Union, 9 May 2008, O.J. (C 115) 13, art. 2 and 3 [hereinafter TEU], Consolidated Version of the Treaty on the Functioning of the European Union, 9 May 2008, O.J. (C 115) 47 [hereinafter TFEU], art. 26 (2); Chalmers et al., 2010). While the free movement between the member states of goods, persons and capital are important in relation to the provision of health care throughout the EU and for the relevant secondary legislation, it is the freedom to provide and receive services that has been central to the development of the law pertaining to cross-border health care. Specifically, Article 56 of the Treaty on the Functioning of the European Union (TFEU)[1] prohibits restrictions on the freedom to provide cross-border services. The European Court of Justice (ECJ) held that, as a natural corollary, this prohibition was also applicable to restrictions on the freedom to receive services (Cohen, 2014; Cases 286/82 and 26/83, *Luisi* v *Ministero Del Tesoro*, 1984).

The ECJ (now renamed the Court of Justice of the European Union, but I will stick with the more traditional abbreviation) has interpreted Article 56 and secondary legislation (specifically Regulation 1408/71, later superseded by Regulation 883/2004 (Regulation 1408/71 of the Council of 14 June 1971 on the Application of Social Security Schemes to Employed Persons and their Families Moving Within the Community 1971 O.J. (L 149) 2 [hereinafter Regulation 1408/71]; Regulation 883/2004, of the European Parliament and of the Council of 29 April 2004 on the Co-ordination of Social Security Systems 2004 O.J. (L 200) 1 [hereinafter Regulation 883/2004]) in its jurisprudence on medical tourism. The ECJ's multiple-decades-long case law on the subject is extensive and complex, and I and others have documented it elsewhere (Cohen, 2014 Quinn and de Hert, 2012; Hatzopolous and Hervey, 2012). In this small space, I will instead jump ahead to 2011, when the EU put into law EU Directive 2011/24 (hereinafter 'The Directive'), which purports to facilitate cross-border health care in the EU, primarily in regard to the 'scheduled care' case rather than 'emergency care' (European Parliament, 2011).

The Directive recognises that EU member states have exclusive responsibility for the organisation and delivery of health care (European Parliament, 2011,

---

1 For the sake of simplicity I will refer to TFEU and the EU rather than their predecessor's treaties and institutions, even when doing so is slightly anachronistic.

Recitals (10), (33), (35) and (64)). The Directive takes into consideration the 'operating principles' that are shared by health systems throughout the Union, and are necessary to ensure patients' trust in cross-border health care and to achieving patient mobility (European Parliament, 2011, Recital (5)). Member states are required to 'transpose' (that is, put into effect) the Directive by 25 October 2013 (European Parliament, 2011, art. 21), and will likely do so in heterogeneous ways, such that it will be some time before we can fully evaluate the scheme.

The Directive is applicable to the provision of health care, 'regardless of how it is organised, delivered and financed' (European Parliament, 2011, art. 1(2)). Health care is defined as 'health services provided by health professionals to patients to assess, maintain or restore their state of health, including the prescription, dispensation and provision of medicinal products and medical devices' (European Parliament, 2011, art. 3(a)). The Directive is inapplicable to long-term care services that are aimed at supporting people in need of assistance in carrying out everyday tasks, as well as the allocation of and access to organs for the purpose of organ transplants, although it does appear to govern the reimbursement of surgical *costs* for these transplants (European Parliament, 2011, art. 1(3)(a) and (b)).

The Directive focuses on four topics: prior authorisation, reimbursement, patient rights and cooperation, but in this short space I will focus only on the first two. Firstly, *prior authorisation schemes*: The Member State of Affiliation is permitted to impose a pre-treatment requirement as a condition of reimbursement for medical tourism, if it would require the same pre-treatment procedure to reimburse the same patient within its territory (European Parliament, 2011, art. 7(7); Quinn and de Hert, 2012, p. 48).

The Directive recognises that the Member State 'of Affiliation may provide for a system of prior authorisation', but in accord with the prior ECJ case law it recognises that such a prior authorisation system can serve as a barrier to the freedom to provide medical services. Therefore, following the ECJ case law, the Directive requires that prior authorisation must be justified and restricted to what is necessary and proportionate to the objective to be achieved (for example, financial balance of social security budget, needs for planning and so on), and may not constitute a means of arbitrary discrimination or unjustified obstacle to the free movement of patients (European Parliament, 2011 art. 8(1); Cohen, 2014).

The Directive specifies both the type of conditions that may justify the establishment of a system of prior authorisation – wherein a Member State of Affiliation requires prior approval before it will pay for medical tourism to a Member State of Treatment – as well as the reasons that have to be met in order to make a refusal of the authorisation lawful. (European Parliament, 2011 art. 8(2), (6)). In terms of the first, the Directive provides that prior authorisation is limited to health care which:

  a) is made subject to planning requirements relating to the object of ensuring
     sufficient and permanent access to a balanced range of high-quality treatment

in the Member State concerned or to the wish to control costs and avoid, as far as possible, any waste of financial, technical and human resources and:

    i) involves overnight hospital accommodation of the patient in question for at least one night; or,

    ii) requires use of highly specialised and cost-intensive medical infrastructure or medical equipment;

b) involves treatments presenting a particular risk for the patient or the population; or,

c) is provided by a healthcare provider that, on a case-by-case basis, could give rise to serious and specific concerns relating to the quality or safety of the care, with the exception of healthcare which is subject to Union legislation ensuring a minimum level of safety and quality throughout the Union.

    (European Parliament, 2011, art. 8(2)).

The Directive embraces the concern raised by the member states as to the effect that unrestricted medical tourism would have on their budget and health policy planning, by providing that prior authorisation requirements may be put in place for non-hospital overnight care that nonetheless requires highly specialised equipment. Additionally, under the Directive, member states will have to provide the Commission a listing of the categories of health care they determine are subject to these planning requirements (European Parliament, 2011, art. 8(2)).

As constructed by the Directive, these categories for which prior authorisation is allowed leave member states with considerable room to manoeuvre. For example, it gives member states latitude in deciding what constitutes major medical equipment in a way that reflects the budgetary constraints of individual member states. The language regarding 'particular risk for the patient or the population' allows member states of Affiliation to require authorisation for those with drug resistant TB or other highly infectious diseases to travel, as well as for those whose unstable condition makes medical tourism a risk to their own health (Quinn and de Hert, 2012, p. 56). The language regarding 'quality or safety of care' may prove the most malleable, since it enables the Member State of Affiliation to apply prior authorisation requirements whenever it is 'concerned' that the foreign care is less safe or efficacious, except in cases where the service in question 'is subject to Union legislation ensuring a minimum level of safety and quality throughout the Union' (Cohen, 2014).

In cases where prior authorisation is used, Article 8(6) of the Directive provides that the Member State of Affiliation may refuse to grant its prior authorisation if:

a) the patient will, according to a clinical evaluation, be exposed with reasonable certainty to a patient-safety risk that cannot be regarded as acceptable, taking into account the potential benefit for the patient of the sought cross-border healthcare;

b) the general public will be exposed with reasonable certainty to a substantial safety hazard as a result of the cross-border healthcare in question;

c) this healthcare is to be provided by a healthcare provider that raises serious and specific concerns relating to the respect of standards and guidelines on quality of care and patient safety, including provisions on supervision, whether these standards and guidelines are laid down by laws and regulations or through accreditation systems established by the Member State of treatment;

d) this healthcare can be provided on its territory within a time limit which is medically justifiable, taking into account the current state of health and the probable course of the illness of each patient concerned.

(European Parliament, 2011 art. 8(6))

On the question of *reimbursement* (Art. 7 of Directive), the second of four topics focused upon, the Directive again mostly accepts and reflects the ECJ case law. The costs of the service provided in the Member State of Treatment will be reimbursed or paid directly by the home Member States of Affiliation 'up to the level of costs that would have been assumed by the [home] state, had this healthcare been provided in its territory' (European Parliament, 2011, art. 7(4), 8(2); Cohen, 2014).

Under the Directive, in cases '[w]here the full cost of cross-border healthcare exceeds the level of costs that would have been assumed had the healthcare been provided in its territory', the Member State of Affiliation retains discretion to 'top up' its reimbursement to make up the difference but is not required to do so. Similarly, it is permitted, but not required, to decide to 'reimburse other related costs, such as accommodation and travel costs, or extra costs which persons with disabilities might incur due to one or more disabilities when receiving' care in the destination country, although as the ECJ noted in the Watts case, such costs should be reimbursed where those costs are normally covered as part of treatment in the Member State of Affiliation of the patient. (European Parliament, 2011, art. 7(4); Cohen, 2014). The Directive also requires that the member state develop 'objective, non-discriminatory criteria known in advance and applied at the relevant (local, regional or national) administrative level' for calculating the amount of reimbursement the Member State of Affiliation will provide (European Parliament, 2011, art. 7(6)).

In fact, the Directive applies its non-discrimination provisions asymmetrically on the Member States of Affiliation and Treatment. The Directive 'encourages but does not oblige member states to adopt legislation ensuring that patients who have availed themselves of the opportunities under the [Directive] for cross-border treatment are entitled to the same rights as if they had opted for treatment in' the Member State of Affiliation. (European Parliament, 2011, art. 7(5), 8(2)). However, as Quinn and de Hert observe, it may be illegal for the Member State of Affiliation to discriminate at home against individuals who had previously used medical tourism in another member state (Quinn and De Hert, 2012, p. 50).

By contrast, discrimination by the Member State of Treatment is explicitly prohibited by the Directive. In particular, while, to the extent permitted by their national health care system, providers in the Member State of Treatment are free to set their own fees, they are prohibited from charging differential rates to medical tourists (European Parliament, 2011, art. 4(4); Quinn and de Hert, 2012, p. 58). The motivation for this rule was apparently the fear that 'if such a requirement were not in place, there would be little to stop providers setting lower prices for residents of other Member States in order to attract non-resident patients ... "crowding out" the market for resident patients' (Quinn and de Hert, 2012, p. 58).

The Directive is a welcome codification and clarification of a tangled ECJ jurisprudence. It is, however, too early to see whether it will significantly facilitate medical tourism within the EU, and as I and others have detailed elsewhere despite its many clarifications the Directive still leaves significant questions unresolved (Cohen, 2014).

Conclusion

Even when it involves only services legal in both the home and destination countries, medical tourism raises a large number of legal and ethical issues. Here I have focused on four. For US patients, the main issues I have discussed are the availability of information about and regulation of the quality of care of foreign hospitals and providers, the risk of deficient medical malpractice recovery, and the regulation of private insurance products incorporating medical tourism. In Europe, where much of the trade is within the EU and home countries have public insurance programmes, the main issues are the legality of prior authorisation schemes and the regulation of reimbursement rates. When it comes to regulation, with their new EU directive, the Europeans are far ahead of the Americans, but in the US state of California, in particular, we have seen some far-sighted regulatory experiments. In this chapter I have tried to lay a path as to where I would like to see the regulation of medical tourism go in other states and at the federal level.

References

Baker, D. and Rho, H.J., 2009. *Free Trade in Health Care: The gains from globalized Medicare and Medicaid.* Washington: Center for Economic Policy and Research. Available at: <http://www.cepr.net/documents/publications/free-trade-hc-2009-09.pdf.> [Accessed 29 December 2013].

Chalmers, D., Davies, G. and Monti, G., 2010. *European Union Law.* Cambridge: Cambridge University Press.

Chandra, A. and Skinner, J., 2004. Geography and Racial Health Disparities. In: N.N. Anderson, R.A. Bulatao and B. Cohen, eds. 2004. *Critical Perspectives on Racial and Ethnic Differences in Late Life.* Washington, DC: National Academies Press, ch. 16.

Cohen, I.G., 2010a. Medical Tourism: The view from ten thousand feet. *Hastings Center Report*, 40(2), pp. 11–12.

————, 2010b. Protecting Patients with Passports: Medical tourism and the patient-protective argument. *Iowa Law Review*, 95(5), pp. 1,467–567.

————, 2012a. How to Regulate Medical Tourism (And Why Bioethicists Should Care). *Journal of Developing World Bioethics*, 12(1), pp. 9–20.

————, 2013. Introduction. In: I.G. Cohen, ed. *The Globalization of Health Care: Legal and ethical challenge*. Oxford: Oxford University Press. Introduction.

————, 2014. *Patients with Passports: Medical tourism, law and ethics*. Oxford: Oxford University Press.

Cortez, N., 2008. Patients without Borders: The emerging global market for patients and the evolution of modern health care. *Indiana Law Journal*, 83, pp. 71–132.

————, 2010. Recalibrating the Legal Risks of Cross-Border Health Care. *Yale Journal of Health Policy, Law, and Ethics*, 10, pp. 1–89.

————, 2011. Embracing the New Geography of Health Care: A novel way to cover those left out of health reform. *Southern California Law Review*, 84, pp. 859–931.

Currie, J. and MacLeod, W.B., 2008. First Do No Harm? Tort reform and birth outcomes. *Quarterly Journal of Economics*, 123(2), pp. 795–830.

Cutler, D., Huckman, R. and Landrum, M., 2004. The Role of Information in Medical Markets: An analysis of publicly reported outcomes in cardiac surgery. *American Economic Review*, 94(2), pp. 342–6.

Ehrbeck, T., Guevara, C. and Mango, P., 2008. Mapping the Market for Medical Travel. *McKinsey Quarterly*, May, pp. 1–8.

Einhorn, B., 2008. Hannaford's Medical-Tourism Experiment. *Business Week*, 9 November.

European Parliament., 2011. Directive 2011/24 of the European Parliament and of the Council of 9 March 2011 on the Application of Patients' Rights in Cross-Border Healthcare. *Official Journal of the European Union*, 88/45.

Flear, M., 2007. Developing Euro-Biocitizens Through Migration for Healthcare Services. *Maastricht Journal of European and Comparative Law*, 14(3), pp. 239–62.

Frakes, M., 2012. Does Medical Malpractice Deter? The impact of tort reforms and malpractice standard reforms on healthcare quality. *Cornell Legal Studies Research Paper*, no. 12–29.

Frank, R., 2004. *Behavioral Economics and Health Economics*. National Bureau of Economic Research. Working Paper no. 10881. Available at: http://www.nber.org/papers/ w10881 [Accessed 29 December 2013].

Greenberg, M., Haviland, A., Ashwood, J.S. and Main, R., 2010. *Is Better Patient Safety Associated with Less Malpractice Activity? Evidence from California*. Sanata Monica: RAND Corporation. Available at: http://www.rand.org/pubs/technical_reports /TR824.html [Accessed 29 December 2013].

Hatzopoulos, V. and Hervey, T., 2012. Coming into Line: The EU's court softens on cross-border health care. *Health Economics, Policy and Law*, 10(1), pp. 1–5.

Herring, B., 2010. Suboptimal Provision of Preventive Healthcare Due to Expected Enrollee Turnover Among Private Insurers. *Health Economics*, 19(4), pp. 438–8.

Lancaster, J., 2004. Surgeries, Side Trips for 'Medical Tourists'. *The Washington Post*, 23 October, p. 1a.

Luisi v *Ministero Del Tesoro*, 1984. E.C.R. 00377.

Madison, K., 2007. Regulating Health Care Quality in an Information Age. *University of California, Davis Law Review*, 40, pp. 1,577–654.

Mattoo, A. and Rathindran, R., 2006. How Health Insurance Inhibits Trade in Health Care. *Health Affairs*, 25(2), pp. 358–68.

Milstein, A. and Smith, M., 2006. America's New Refugees – Seeking affordable surgery offshore. *New England Journal of Medicine*, 355(16), pp. 1,637–40.

Murphy, T., 2009. Health Insurers Explore Savings in Overseas Care. *Associated Press*, 23 August.

Quinn, P. and de Hert, P., 2012. The European Patients' Rights Directive: A clarification and codification of individual rights relating to cross border healthcare and novel initiatives aimed at improve pan-European healthcare cooperation. *Medical Law International*, 12(1), pp. 28–69.

Sawicki, N., 2012. Patient Protection and Decision-Aid Quality: Regulatory and tort law approaches. *Arizona Law Review*, 54, pp. 621–72.

Schneider, C. and Hall, M., 2009. The Patient Life: Can consumers direct health care? *American Journal of Law and Medicine*, 35, pp. 7–66.

The Kaiser Family Foundation and Agency for Health Care Research and Quality, 2002. *National Survey on Americans as Health Care Consumers: An update on the role of quality information*. Washington, DC: The Henry J. Kaiser Family Foundation. Available at: http://www.ahrq.gov/downloads/pub/ kffchartbk00.pdf. [Accessed 29 December 2013].

Turner, L. 2013. Patient Mortality in Medical Tourism: Examining news media reports of deaths following travel for cosmetic surgery and bariatric surgery. In: I.G. Cohen, ed. *The Globalization of Health Care: Legal and ethical challenge*. Oxford: Oxford University Press, ch. 1.

Wallace, S., Mendez-Luck, C. and Castañeda, X., 2009. Heading South: Why Mexican immigrants in California seek health services in Mexico. *Medical Care*, 47(6), pp. 662–9.

Chapter 11

Race to the Bottom or Race to the Top? Governing Medical Tourism in a Globalised World

Ingrid Schneider

Introduction

Medical tourism as a burgeoning phenomenon is both an effect and an expression of globalisation processes. The growth of international trade and markets, touristic infrastructures, acceleration, mobility and flexibility, communication facilitated through the internet, together with the sometimes aggressive marketing of respective 'services' have contributed to a striking rise in cross-border health care. Medical tourism has gained political support, both within Europe and beyond, not least within policy programmes to create a European single market and in the context of international trade agreements. Medical tourism is predominately sailing under the banner of economic justification. It does so by highlighting the comparative cost advantages if medical services can be provided elsewhere more cost-effectively and with possibly even higher standards of care. Medical tourism has become big business, a multi-billion dollar industry with hospitals competing for hundreds of thousands of patients who are travelling to obtain medical care across the world every year (Lunt et al., 2012a).

The main question of this chapter is: how can medical tourism be governed in a globalised world? The response is structured in several parts: first, after a short definition, some push and pull factors for medical tourism are presented. Second, instances and tools which pertain to horizontal and vertical forms of regulatory governance of medical tourism are analysed. Third, the question of whether medical tourism incites a race to the bottom or a race to the top in terms of ethical and socio-economic standards of health care will be discussed. In this context, normative questions arise, for instance whether and how to sanction the purposeful evasion of domestic laws. Discursive practices of governance also matter, such as how the framing of the issues impacts on the regulatory solutions sought. Furthermore there is the issue of moral pluralism and how it can be dealt with without relapsing into moral relativism or even moral nihilism. Each of these elements informs a conclusion regarding the extent to which we can secure high standards and good practices of medical care and, thus, better global governance of medical tourism.

Governance research within political science investigates how individuals or organisations structure their actions which, in sum, coordinate activities to solve collective problems. According to this broad definition, governance is an overarching term, comprising both government and governance. Hence, this analytical perspective combines traditional concepts of vertical governance, in which the state (by 'command and control') regulates public functions and implements collectively binding decisions from the 'top down', with complementary processes of horizontal governance. Horizontal governance implies self-regulation through networks of public, private and civil society actors. Therefore, in the following, the term 'governance' is understood in a process-oriented perspective, employing an institutionalist approach which is an extension of classical steering theories, following the works of Mayntz and Scharpf (Mayntz, 1998). Governance deals with regulatory structures, combining public and private, state as well as market, hierarchical and networked forms of action coordination. According to this actor-centred institutionalist governance theory, actions taken by individuals or collective actors operate 'in the shadow of hierarchy' (a term coined by Fritz Scharpf, 1997) cast by state agencies that mediate processes of 'regulated self-regulation' even if the state does not intervene directly. Hence, governance provides a theoretical framework for analysing which regulatory variables favour or disfavour medical tourism, and which have an influence on how medical tourism is being performed.

Medical Tourism: Push and Pull Factors

'Medical tourism' covers a wide range of heterogeneous practices. It is a fuzzy term that is hard to define and different types of medical tourism can be distinguished. The first simply relates to patients travelling to a foreign country to obtain medical care. The second definition includes the recruitment and migration of medical doctors and nurses as well as medical researchers to countries where there is better payment or more favourable conditions for work and scientific activities. A third extended definition involves the shipment not only of drugs and medical products but also of bodily substances such as blood, sperm or oocytes from one state to another. A fourth type involves the outsourcing of medical trials to the global South. A fifth extends to highly experimental medical therapies, such as medical tourists travelling in search of stem cell treatments to China and yet another explores whether medical care sought abroad is legal in the patient's home country or whether it is contrary to national law (Cohen, 2010). The latter refers for instance to oocyte donation or Preimplantation Genetic Diagnosis (PGD) in several European countries, or to doctor-assisted suicide ('euthanasia tourism') in Switzerland. Especially problematic are cases in which medical tourism is offered for services which are unlawful both in the home and in the destination country, such as the organ trade. Particularly thorny legal and ethical questions about proxy consent and admissibility are raised for minors, such as sick children whose parents travel with them to foreign destinations, and even more so if this is done for purposes of experimental medical therapy. Moreover, special challenges arise when cross-border reproductive tourism involves gametes or reproductive services (surrogacy) that necessitate the involvement of a third party, as this involves not only the patient–doctor relationship, but invokes issues of genealogy, kinship, triangles or quadrangles of biological and social relationships, and as such touches directly upon the interests and putative rights of the child-to-be (Schneider, 2003). This contribution will mainly refer to the first mentioned, narrow type of medical tourism. However, it will also tackle some of the normative and legal issues involved in the latter types.

With respect to governance, we may depart from the perspective that medical tourism is, in its most general form, an effect of differences and divergences in health care, laws, economics and socio-cultural practices. Analytically, we can divide between push and pull factors for medical tourism:

- **Push factors** include the lack of health care or dissatisfaction with medical services in the home country. Among the factors pushing patients abroad are frustration with the health care system due to prolonged waiting periods, insufficient insurance coverage, the unavailability of treatments due to limitations imposed by governmental agencies or insurers, the lack of advanced treatment facilities or limited specialist care or the lack of trust in the quality of doctors and medical services provided;
- **Pull factors** for seeking diagnostic or therapeutic treatment abroad comprise time, cost, and quality considerations, such as lower costs of care, price savings, faster availability of specialist care, but also at times higher quality of medical personnel or the availability of cutting-edge experimental treatments (Lunt et al., 2011; Lunt et al., 2012b; Crooks et al., 2010).

As a next step, I analyse the most important regulatory institutions which influence the decisions of patients to travel abroad. Systematically considering these regulatory instruments may also identify sites for interventions, such as tools and levers to either increase or decrease the demand for cross-border medical care. We will start with horizontal forms of governance. In the following, some regulatory variables will be discussed which include the actions of health care insurers, the medical community, networks of researchers and the media.

Variables in the Horizontal Governance of Medical Tourism

Cost Coverage by Health Insurance or National Health Care System

Whether or not the public health service or a patient's health insurance covers elective medical care provided in another country is a key factor for the behaviour of patients. If medical treatment in the destination country is reimbursed by the insurer this provides a welcome opportunity for patients to bypass restrictions perceived in the home country. In some cases, health insurance funds will even direct their insurance holders to hospitals abroad with whom they hold agreements on discounts for the optional services in question. But as insurers will not refund each and every thing, the conditions imposed on cost coverage for foreign medical services are crucial. In this respect, it makes a big difference whether certification of foreign hospitals is called for, whether insurer and medical care providers have to sign anterior contracts or whether prior approved estimations of costs are demanded. Even when patients pay out of their own pocket for health care administered in another country, it will be of paramount importance to them whether their health insurance covers payment for necessary follow-up care.

This holds true not only for regular supervision of progress in health status, but also for costly expenses normally covered by health insurers such as the payment of regular immunosuppressive drugs after organ transplantation (a situation that may escalate when it pertains to the treatment of adverse effects of medical services administered abroad). The degree to which foreign clinics can issue contractual waivers for complications and unexpected but necessary follow-up care may vary, and so does the spectre of follow-up treatments which the domestic health care system and private or public insurers are willing to provide, and to pay for. Such legal, financial and other barriers may be elevated if it relates to highly experimental remedies prescribed abroad or if the treatment given was illegal in the patient's home country. Israel, for instance, in its 2008 Organ Transplant Act, has prohibited reimbursement for foreign organ transplants if those organs were purchased in another state, such as China, where transplanted organs come from executed prisoners (Keller, 2013).

Proving medical malpractice will always be a difficult undertaking, even more so if it happened in another country. However, the importance of cost coverage can also generate a tool by which to influence foreign standards of care; if health insurers were capable of imposing conditions upon foreign doctors or health care centres they could improve the quality of care, prevent unskilful medical treatments and also foster recovery from medical malpractice. They may even prohibit a contractual waiver of medical malpractice thereby enforcing duties on physicians and clinics. Providing respective *information* to patients to allow them to make informed choices is another instrument available for steering patients' actions, thus turning health insurers and/or national health providers into key agents for regulating patients' demands for cross-border care. In the same vein, the potentials and limits of *contract law* between domestic and foreign health care providers must be emphasised as levers for policing medical tourism.

Liability Law

In a closely related way, the 'ifs and hows' of liability for complications arising from medical treatments abroad are another important regulatory factor in cross-border medical care. However, rules about the onus of proof for ill health or medical malpractice are tricky legal questions. It can be very difficult to prove that medical complications are caused by the wrongful actions of medical doctors, as it is not always easy to establish that a mistake or negligence has occurred. This process becomes more arduous if different layers of legal regimes and several jurisdictions have to be taken into account. Many questions about the potential and limits of contractual agreements and liability remain unsettled. Can risks and adverse reactions be controlled via liability law? How can foreign providers be held accountable for adverse effects or malpractices? How far can the onus of proof for medical malpractice be inversed from patient to physician? In such circumstances the regulatory state may have to step in, raising further issues and questions: what role can patient protection laws, legal and social counselling services, ombudspersons at clinics or public agencies play in providing support should problems occur? How important will documentation requirements and registers – who was treated when, by whom and how? – be as evidence-protection measures that can provide indications of liability in case of malpractice suits, ill health or other negative consequences of foreign health care.

Liability law is a terrain in which the inextricable interaction between private, contractual, public, regulatory as well as administrative law comes to the fore.[1] In all of these lamentable cases, a lot of money will be needed for attorneys, courts and lawyers in general. Such expenses may sum up to considerable amounts. From a macro-economic perspective, it is questionable whether, if such costs were included in cost-benefit assessment, increased public spending for domestic health care would not provide a better option for providing effective health care to citizens.

Self-Regulation of the Medical Community

Medical associations are powerful organisations, as they combine authoritative expert knowledge with professional honours, traditions and privileges. As professional federations they have special principles and codes of conduct such as professional guidelines, rules of best practice, and proper legal means of sanctioning the members of the guild at their command. Whether medical associations recommend or outlaw certain forms of medical tourism will certainly impact upon such practices. Public memoranda or policy papers published by medical associations attract attention and do have an influence on legislation and insurers alike. Individual physicians and specialist societies representing medical

---

1 Private law is that part of a civil law legal system which involves relationships between individuals, such as the law of contracts or torts, and the law of obligations. It is to be distinguished from public law, which deals with relationships between both persons or organisations and the state, including regulatory statutes, penal law and other law that affects the public order. In general terms, private law involves interactions between private citizens and private parties, whereas public law involves interrelations between the state and the general population.

fields can provide an important contribution when it comes to counselling for or against medical tourism. As general practitioners and family doctors may have a particularly long and trusting relationship with their patients, their voice and advice will exert a special authority. Medical associations can do a lot to support their members in providing these counselling activities by providing relevant information to them. In Canada, for instance, doctors are provided with information about the risks of stem cell tourism (Caulfield and Condit, 2012).

Even if most medical associations are national organisations, there are also forums for transnational, regional and international agreement among physicians and health professionals. Debating medical tourism at international conferences, drafting guidelines of professional conduct, setting standards for best practices and passing codes of ethics do play important normative roles in establishing what is permissible in cross-border health care. Even if such 'soft law' cannot legally be enforced on an international scale, it will have an impact on regulating medical practices, not least in educating doctors' consciences. Normative claims and demands by peers may, to a certain degree, counteract solely profit-driven behaviour. At least it will provide norms for 'naming and shaming' as well-known governance practices – be it of individual doctors, medical centres or even countries – that do not comply with these professional norms. As an example, the Declaration of Istanbul on Organ Trafficking and Transplant Tourism, which condemned transplant tourism and commercial markets for human organs (Delmonico, 2009), has reinforced the universal norm of non-commodification of the human body. Even though such statements will not stop trade in organs altogether, they have deterred states (except Iran, and to a certain extent Israel) from adopting regulated market schemes for organ transplantation from living donors (Schneider, 2014). Thus, the outlawing of certain practices by the medical community and physicians speaking out and taking action within and beyond their jurisdiction may help close legal loopholes and create an environment in which abusive practices cannot flourish. Physicians have demanded from society a large degree of autonomy over their professional acts, including the freedom to treat patients according to their best judgment, and this has played a key role in how doctors have defined themselves as professionals historically. Today, it remains important to remind them about the responsibilities stemming from these rights, particularly that rights to self-regulation must be coupled with respective duties. In this respect, some medical paternalism is certainly justified when it comes to warning patients about the risks associated with medical tourism (O'Neill, 2002).

Researchers' Communities

In a similar way to physicians, researchers have also long crossed national borders to acquire knowledge and to undertake collaborative work. Peer review plays an extraordinarily important role not only in scientific publication, but also in assessing the quality of professional work performed by other researchers. Reputation is, thus, a crucial currency in science. Similarly to medical associations, scientific researchers have an obligation and duty not to overhype the potentially therapeutic results of innovative research. Networks, for instance of stem cell scientists, must tackle scientific malpractice and respond to misrepresentations of therapeutic promise by colleagues in their own or foreign countries or in the media. In this respect they have a responsibility to increase the publics' and politicians' sensitivity to health risks associated with new medical technologies and not fall prey to illusions and (self-)deceptions about speedy development or magical cures; particularly so, if such promises are driven by self-serving motives. Desperate people seeking desperate measures have to be protected from harm and exploitation by reckless researchers performing premature clinical trials, and from rush-to-profit clinical entities offering unproven treatments (Magnus and Cho, 2007). Parts of the research community have long recognised that promising too much too early creates expectations that cannot be met by real science and will thus foster a backlash impacting on good scientific practices and legitimate research. It is their task to stop colleagues from selling bad science or raising unrealistic expectations. Institutional support for whistleblowing, diligent peer review and institutional measures to avoid and prevent conflicts of interests may counter unfounded excitement and the overhyping of new medical technologies.

Media Representations

The way the media frames and represents medical research, treatment and medical tourism also has an impact upon patients' perceptions. This relates to news media and to social media alike. There may be a general media bias towards the hopeful human-interest story, one about surprising survival and unexpected cure, at the expense of the cautionary tale. Many observers have suggested that '-omics' research is often inappropriately hyped in both the popular media and the scientific literature evoking the very-near prospect of future cures (Bubela and Caulfield, 2004). This hype has the potential to create a range of social concerns and can even add to a vicious circle of hope and hype, with detrimental societal effects. Some have termed this complex array of social forces a 'hype pipeline', constructed by a combination of: pressure upon scientists to publish; intense commercialisation agendas aimed at maximising profits, jobs and economic growth by quickly translating scientific research from bench to bedside; the filing of patents; and the generation of hyperbolic messages emanating from universities as well as funding institutions, the news media and even from the public itself (Caulfield and Condit, 2012).

These numerous interrelated factors can only be countered by utilising a wide range of policy strategies. Among these are those which call for the self-regulation of journalists, media and even bloggers. Publishing houses, editors and media associations can often reach out to fellow journalists in workshops and other forums to educate them about responsible scientific journalism. This may help the public to understand that science is a slow, iterative process with necessary failures. The media can highlight that medical progress may not yet benefit current patients – only future generations – and also help expose bogus experimental 'therapies'.

Another function that the media can perform is to report on the dark sides of medical tourism, particularly those associated with exploitative practices and with the abuse of people and their bodies in foreign countries. As patient demand is one of the driving forces for medical tourism, and as social media has become influential in spreading the word about treatment opportunities elsewhere, it seems appropriate that such outlets also provide more transparency about their sources. Foreign clinics and pharmaceutical companies often actively involve patients in their marketing strategies through social media and patient platforms. Doctors, civic education services and patient support groups must make clear that information drawn from such sources is self-interested and biased. More trustworthy independent sources of information that can provide more objective knowledge and clinical evidence on proven efficacy are much needed and have to be supported by the State. Boosting public literacy about current research frameworks, the risks and ambiguities of medical progress, and the socio-economic conditions in which medical innovation is taking place may provide an important antidote to over-selling and hype whilst also moderating patients' demand for foreign treatment. The governance mechanisms discussed so far largely rely on forms of professional self-regulation and on regulation within functional systems of society, sometimes supported by regulated self-regulation. The next section is dedicated to highlighting the importance of public intervention by state agencies.

Vertical Governance of Medical Tourism: Public Policy, Law and Courts

Targeting medical tourism through public policy measures is a complex field. Some destination countries such as Thailand, the Philippines, Singapore and Malaysia, invest heavily in offering appealing sites for medical tourists and in providing the necessary infrastructure for making medical tourism flourish (Pocock and Phua, 2011). Emerging countries like India and Brazil fund extravagant health care facilities to create lucrative 'hubs' designed to increase patient traffic, revenue and thus foreign exchange earnings. Some Southern and Eastern European countries also place emphasis on the medical tourism industry in the hope of stimulating their national economy. Poland, the Czech Republic and Hungary have become important destinations for dentistry and cosmetic surgery, Spain and Cyprus for fertility tourism and Turkey for organ transplantation. Even in Northern European countries such as Germany or Belgium, filling private hospital beds with affluent citizens from Middle Eastern countries (and adjacent hotel suites with their family members) has become a strategy that has pleased shareholders (Kulish and Cottrell, 2012). Therefore, it is reasonable to assume that medical tourism will gain further momentum. Of course, one must not condemn each and every form of medical tourism. If it were only for the specialist treatment of rare diseases or for hip replacement and dental care there would be little to object to in patients crossing borders when high quality can be secured. Citizens seeking services abroad may also imply that services are insufficient in quantity, type, timing or affordability in the home country. It may thus provide a valuable prompt for the departure country to improve the quality and accessibility of domestic health services. However, when it comes to cosmetic surgery, fertility or organ tourism, not to mention euthanasia tourism, the stakes are much higher as far as the moral and social costs are concerned.

The growth of medical tourism generally may be an alarming trend as it raises a number of concerns. In socio-economic terms, such practices may reinforce economic disparities and exacerbate health inequalities within and between states. They may arguably create a bifurcation of care for foreign and domestic patients, to the detriment of the latter. In general, they may create a global misallocation of health resources, infrastructure and personnel (de Arellano, 2007). Key issues in this respect are the brain-drain of well-trained medical doctors and nurses to wealthy hospitals and limited access to health care for less well-off patients. Patients travelling abroad may also have negative effects on the costs and availability of domestic health care, as where options for treatment exist abroad, countries lacking good and timely medical services may feel little pressure to address domestic shortages. Patients from countries with strong, publicly-funded health care systems who are seeking cross-border medical care subtly undermine the underlying public ethos of such national health systems. In effect, a second tier of care is being introduced which is available only to those with the ability to pay; this runs contrary to the ideal of universal coverage of publicly-funded health care and the conception that health care should be allocated according to need and should not be treated as a commodity. In both departure and destination countries, medical tourism may thus work to neutralise pressures for reform and for the equitable distribution of resources (Crooks et al., 2010).

In sum, medical tourism may neither alleviate poverty nor be supportive for building a functional national health system for the benefit of all (Tattara, 2010). There is, as yet, insufficient systematic evidence about the aggregate benefits and losses to conclusively state whether medical tourism 'is virus, symptom, or cure' (Lunt et al., 2011, p. 44), though this does substantiate calls for further exploration and empirical research (Crooks et al., 2010; Johnston et al., 2010). However, even when evidence is inconclusive, regulation is still needed and policy-makers are called upon to act.

Criminal Law

When it comes to issues of legal jurisdictions, the *territoriality* of law is confronted with the *extraterritoriality* of the services provided. In liberal market democracies, the State will not and cannot prohibit its citizens from travelling abroad to choose health care. Criminal law can only be a response if serious harm has been inflicted – whether on national citizens or on patients from abroad – and laws have been violated, How far law enforcement can be extended across national borders remains a difficult question in international criminal law. One possible model for extraterritorial regulation is that of sex tourism with minors. In these cases, states such as the US and Germany have passed extra-territorial legislation allowing them to carry out investigations, prosecute and punish any individual guilty of crimes committed abroad and linked to child sex abuse (Cohen, 2010, p. 11). However, criminal penalties for more-or-less-desperate patients who have sought remedies for their conditions through the illegal organ trade can only be a measure of *ultima ratio*; as in many jurisdictions laws exempt patients from such penalties.

Civil and Administrative Law

In contrast, civil law can possibly provide some means to deter people from certain cross-border activities. Such has been the case in several instances regarding couples from Norway, Germany and Italy who had sought surrogacy services in India. As an example, in early 2008, twins born to an Indian surrogate mother were denied entry to Germany. The German authorities did not issue passports for the infants because surrogate motherhood is prohibited in Germany. In addition, according to German law, the legal mother of a child is the one who has carried it to term. Children born to surrogate mothers overseas on behalf of German 'commissioning parents' do not acquire German citizenship at birth. After the Bavarian couple fought the case through the courts, visas were finally issued in 2010. In another case, a Berlin court ruled in 2010 that a child born to a surrogate mother in India had no right to a German passport despite having a German biological father. Under both German and Indian law, the legal father of a child born by surrogacy is actually the surrogate mother's husband. The biological father in this case was a German citizen. The birth certificate from the Indian hospital recorded the German man and his wife as the parents, but the German embassy in India refused to issue a German passport for the child.

Even if denial of citizenship to a newborn child may be regarded as a harsh dissuasive measure, this may serve as an example of how medical tourism across borders can be regulated. In the Germans case the court decision is seen to fulfil an appellative, law-stabilising function and, thus, a general preventive function, which highlights the values set by the legislature (The Local, 2011). Such cases prompted the Indian state to issue strict visa guidelines and to demand, from 2013, a specific 'medical' visa for commissioning parents travelling to India for surrogacy. Applications are restricted to heterosexual couples, married for at least two years, who must also cite evidence that surrogacy is legal in their home country. Furthermore, they must demonstrate that their home country would recognise the child born of the surrogacy arrangement as their biological child (Hyder, 2013). However, in the case of Germany, two recent High Court decisions may have opposite effects by providing a gateway for legalising children created by foreign surrogacy mothers. One High Court has ruled that embassies must now issue visas for children if the surrogate mother was not married and the sperm donor was the biological father.[2] The Federal Court of Justice has also since ruled that foreign court decisions must be acknowledged if they attribute parenthood to commissioning parents, if one of those parents is a genetic father.[3] What is clear is that visa and citizenship policies, however operationalized, provide important means to govern medical tourism through administrative law.

In a similar manner, national non-anonymity requirements for gamete donors in civil law can also potentially have protective and preventive effects upon choice of foreign gamete donors. The rights of donor-conceived people not to be deceived or deprived of information about their personal history could be protected through such means. As the welfare and best interests of the child imply the right to know about his or her genetic origin, mechanisms for donor registration could be set up and enforced upon other countries. This would enable offspring who wish to know about – and potentially contact – their genetic parent, to have access to the recorded information when they reach age 18. Laws cannot force parents to tell the truth to children, but they can provide instruments to enable donor-conceived offspring to know where they came from if they so wish (Schneider, 2009). Thus, certain practices would not be legally prohibited *per se*, but rather discouraged, while others are actively promoted. In this respect we can clearly see the transition that can occur from imperative law towards creative governance tools that work through incentives and encouragement (Hoffmann-Riem, 2000). At present it is evident that the toolbox for innovative public policy measures to encourage responsible practices has not yet been explored to the full. Furthermore, at this level we still dealing with bilateral or transnational modes of governance. As a next step, international level measures will be outlined as an additional dimension of global governance.

Global Governance by International Conventions, Declarations, Agreements and Courts

International conventions, declarations and agreements on medical tourism would certainly be desirable to provide for high quality care and the maintenance of safety standards as well as for ethical and legal limits to exploitative practices or outright bans thereof. However, such standards and agreements are not easy to obtain. Currently, there is no United Nations organisation engaged in the coordination or delivery of accreditation schemes which would restrict supply, by either approving or licencing medical care providers (Lunt et al., 2011, p. 42). Neither international associations for consumer protection nor health advocacy groups have taken up this issue. In the case of the most controversial practices, however, at least some consensus could be reached.

---

2   Decision by OLG Duesseldorf, 3. Zivilsenat, I-3 WX 211/12, 3 WX 211/12, 26 April 2013.

3   Federal Court of Justice BGH, XII ZB 463/13, 10 December 2014.

Regional law-making, in particular in the European Union, has already achieved some progress. The EU blood directive (2002/98/EC) as well as the requirements introduced by the EU cell and tissue directive (2004/23/EC), have increased safety standards and oversight, and thus can be seen as important steps forward. Additionally, the EU regulations on advanced therapy medicinal products (Directive 2001/83/EC and Regulation (EC) No 1394/2007) as well as the organ transplantation directive (2010/53/EC) have been passed. The main common goals and features of these regulations are high and uniform standards for safety and quality as controlled by public medical authorities. These regulations have contributed to public trust.

As guiding principles they have emphasised altruism, solidarity and non-commercial donation and have also stressed universal values as well as understandings of human rights protections. The European Precautionary Principle requires caution to be practised in the context of uncertainty and states that, in the absence of scientific consensus, that when there is a risk that an action or policy is harmful priority is given to ensuring human health.[4] However, these aforementioned principles and directives have not yet sufficiently addressed the specific issues raised, for example, by the transnational germ cell trade and fertility treatments, or by patient tourism for experimental research. Therefore, further regulation at the EU level is needed.

The Council of Europe is another regional regulator and to date comprises 47 member states. Even though, in contrast to the EU, it cannot make binding laws, it can issue 'soft law' in the form of recommendations and reports. The Council of Europe is currently preparing a convention against trafficking in human organs (Council of Europe, 2012). Once adopted by the Committee of Ministers, it will be the first legally binding international instrument devoted to combatting organ trafficking. It will also consider a road map for an additional protocol against the trafficking of human tissues and cells. The European Court of Human Rights (ECHR) in Strasbourg, which enforces the European Convention on Human Rights, has become another important regulatory institution. It has issued a number of decisions on issues with biomedical relevance. The ECHR has acquired the status of a transnational, pan-European constitutional court (Stone-Sweet, 2011, p. 236).

---

4   The Precautionary Principle is enshrined in paragraph 2 of article 191 of the EU's Lisbon treaty. While a comprehensive definition of the Precautionary Principle was never formally adopted by the EU, Rene von Schomberg proposed the following working definition and implementation strategy for the EU context: 'Where, following an assessment of available scientific information, there are reasonable grounds for concern for the possibility of adverse effects but scientific uncertainty persists, provisional risk management measures based on a broad cost-benefit analysis whereby priority will be given to human health and the environment, necessary to ensure the chosen high level of protection in the Community and proportionate to this level of protection, may be adopted, pending further scientific information for a more comprehensive risk assessment, without having to wait until the reality and seriousness of those adverse effects become fully apparent' (Schomberg in Fisher et al., 2006).

It provides an important focal point for contestations as an application can be brought either by individuals or by one or more contracting states, and, besides judgements, it can also issue advisory opinions.

On the international level regulation by the United Nations could be most powerful if it were passed as an international convention, but even if there were only a non-binding UN declaration this 'soft law' could set some ethical standards and provide for guidance. One example is the UN Declaration on Human Cloning (59/280) which was adopted in 2005 and called upon signatory nations 'to prohibit all forms of human cloning', including both reproductive cloning and research cloning (Somatic Cell Nuclear Transfer).[5] It also called upon members 'to take measures to prevent the exploitation of women in the application of life sciences' (Schneider, 2009).

It is important to highlight that supranational regulation and governance cannot and will not mean uniform standards. It can only provide minimum standards that must be met by all the states that allow certain ethically or socio-economically controversial practices to take place within their respective jurisdictions. This does not prevent any state from maintaining or introducing in its territory more stringent protective measures. It would not undermine domestic regulation prohibiting certain practices if democratic decision-making had come to prefer this means of regulation, but it would provide some protection for vulnerable citizens living under more permissive regimes.

Race to the Bottom or Race to the Top? And what about Moral Pluralism?

Before turning to mid and long-term tendencies in medical tourism, and in particular towards evaluative assessments, a caveat seems to be in order. In the context of governance research, we may point to some ambiguities in current discourses on medical tourism. Governance does not only occur by law and practices but also via language and discursive practices (Schneider, 2010, pp. 71–104). Frequently, descriptive assessments of present developments come along with normative connotations. These descriptive and prescriptive dimensions can only be distinguished analytically, and often they are happily mixed up in talks, debates and even in scholarly articles. In addition, the debate on medical tourism often blends together safety and quality standards with normative rules. This chapter calls for more analytical differentiation.

Much of the literature on cross-border health care contains an underlying assumption, namely that more mobility would favour a tendency towards liberalisation of national laws which regulate biomedical practices. Such a

---

5   An international cloning *convention* could not be achieved. In the meantime, the advancement of induced-pluripotent cells (ips) has rendered most of SCNT research obsolete. This may also provide a lesson for governance: sometimes, new technical achievements can mitigate and supersede value conflicts in the global realm.

liberalisation, so the argument goes, is already the result of moral pluralism in modern liberal and democratic societies anyway. In this context, one may point to more social tolerance and legal equality for children born outside of wedlock; a growing acceptance of homosexuality; an equality of rights between same-sex couples and the traditional family; equal rights for women and men; and the legal and safe provision of abortion, contraception and other sexual and reproductive health care. These emancipatory developments have been fought for by civil rights movements. Crossing borders for respective care has only played a minor role in such moral liberalisation, if any at all.

The case may be more difficult, though, for wicked ethical problems implied by the advent of new technologies, especially in reproduction where more than a single, morally autonomous individual is involved or when interventions at the very beginning or the end of human life are concerned. Therefore, a short excurse: In many democracies, civil society as well as policy-makers have come to the conclusion that doing nothing about regulation is not a viable option, as fundamental societal values and constitutional norms are affected. However, dealing with moral clashes in pluralist societies is a tricky undertaking. In contrast to interest conflicts or to risk conflicts, in value conflicts compromises are hard to achieve. Often fundamental principles are involved, in which there is no 'more or less' but only a 'yes or no' position at hand. Whether, and to what extent, moral conflicts can be resolved by majority rule, as other issues in democratic decision-making are, is also a highly delicate question. Ultimately, responsibility will be placed on the democratic legislator to decide by majority rule, but beforehand there should be extended forums in parliaments and civil society for in-depth deliberation and for societal resolution of deeply dividing conflicts. Even if complete consensus may be illusory, attempts at approximation may lead to reframing of the issues at stake and thus to some overarching common understandings which make legal solutions possible (Schneider, 2010, pp. 91–6, 553–70). In that respect, such moral compromises may sometimes be philosophically inconsistent but legally and socially viable. Such compromises may defuse and appease social conflicts before they become violent.

There is anecdotal evidence to support the liberalisation argument. Strict laws – for instance on PGD or on destructive research on human embryos – have been replaced by more permissive regulation in some countries. Admittedly, the supply and demand for patient tourism generated by globalised health care, economic competition, research races and ambitious national medical tourism programmes may also put some pressure on the deregulation of national laws. Some patient and donor-protective mechanisms or strict normative rules have been repealed in favour of new, liberalised rules.

However, on closer inspection this liberalisation trend is not as unidirectional as it may seem to be. Even though some tendencies towards liberalisation are undeniable, some states have also opted for stricter and more prohibitive regulation, and/or have proven resilient towards hollowing out or abolishing such restrictions. Moreover, liberalisation can even be reversed. For example, in 2003, Italy opted for very restrictive IVF legislation after several decades of quite liberal and unregulated practices when it had become the destination of choice for post-menopausal women undergoing IVF combined with egg donation. Some countries, such as Canada, Germany, Norway, Austria – and to some extent also France and Switzerland – have also maintained relatively strict laws about consumptive research on human embryos as well as on reproductive medicine in general. In conclusion, in the fertility, embryology and gamete donation sector a patchwork of European regulations can be observed (European Commission, 2006) which has not become more uniform but even more diverse in its approaches and in the variety of regulations. Not infrequently, more liberal practices existed without explicit legal regulation until parliamentary legislators stepped in when rules became less permissive. In addition, scandals and scientific fraud cases such as the Hwang Woo-suk cloning case in South Korea in 2006,[6] as well as disclosure of cases of organ trafficking or cases of serious harm inflicted by certain forms of medical tourism, have led to the tightening of the ethical-legal rules heightening the level of the international playing field.

However, there exists also a counterclaim to the liberalisation paradigm: Some discussants argue that medical tourism could work as a 'safety valve', allowing pluralist societies to maintain higher ethical standards while dissatisfied citizens can and will travel abroad. In this view, medical tourism relieves pressure for a change of national legislation. Often, this argument is accompanied by accusations of hypocrisy against states that have passed and maintained prohibitive rules on medical tourism (Pennings, 2002).

Another perspective which is closely related to the liberalisation paradigm assumes a quasi-'natural' race towards lower thresholds: As cheaper services or treatments that are illegal in the source country are offered in other states, patients will 'vote with their feet', hence pick and choose. The underlying assumption here is that there will be a competition for undercutting both normative and legal standards. Therefore, it is postulated that liberal societies under globalisation pressures tend to lower the bar meaning that safety standards will necessarily decline and normative standards will erode as a consequence. In terms of connotation, some celebrate this suggested development as progress towards more and more liberty. Others, from the camp of culture pessimists, complain about the downfall of these civilising accomplishments. A third camp, often religiously associated, decries the decline of moral standards and public order which is frequently expressed in 'slippery slope' metaphors. Yet others argue that competitive races will lead to the constant improvement of standards of care as countries have to compete with others for ever better services as well as for proper and safe normative regulation to attract patients from abroad.

---

6 Hwang Woo-suk was considered one of the world's pioneers in cloning research until it was uncovered that all his scientific articles claiming success in creating human embryonic stem cells by cloning were based on fraud.

More research is needed to assess how these aforementioned hypotheses can be tested and which of them can be maintained after thorough scrutiny. As a preliminary conclusion, it can be argued that neither a 'convergence to the top' nor a 'race to the bottom' fully captures the diverse developments and contradictory tendencies now emerging. This observation underlines the decisive role of political regulation in the competitive downgrading or upgrading of safety, quality and ethical standards in transnational health care. It may even be the case that generalisations of this kind are inadequate. Often such general verdicts are made with a special aspect of cross-border medical care in mind, one not easily transferred to other cases. But even regarding single issues, controversies abound as different framings, understandings and assessments of the case in question are involved.

The most telling examples of the great variances in the framing of cross-border practices involve heterologous insemination by sperm donation, IVF for single women, egg donation for reproductive purposes or for stem cell and SCNT techniques and surrogate motherhood contracts for gay men. The application of all these techniques also implies moral judgements about sexual behaviour, procreation and parenthood. It touches upon the potential of plurality and the limits of tolerance. It is about the balance between societal norms on the one-hand and individual rights and obligations on the other. Some discussants may point to the loosening of the fetters of hetero-normativity and celebrate the final dissociation of sex from procreation. Others may be more sceptical and ask who is paying the price in terms of exploitation of female bodies, labour and reproductive capacities. Another, related perspective stresses the unforeseen physical and psychical risks in such contractual arrangements which may take a toll on the liberty and physical integrity of vulnerable citizens. Another critique highlights the welfare and needs of children born out of such contractual agreements, who may later want to know their genetic or biological origins. For sure, the multiplication of biological, genetic and social parenthood calls for new negotiations about the rights and duties among all those who have contributed to a child's birth and upbringing. How to secure reliable relationships and safe bonding? A trivialisation of parenthood may certainly not be in the best interest of a child-(to-be). As evidenced here in all practices of medical tourism, race, class and gender divisions within and across societies are inextricably involved. Such inequalities and disparities may pose challenges, even if the biomedical practices, as such, were uncontroversial. Even more difficult are practices which may violate social norms.

As yet, it is unclear how value conflicts can be productively dealt with in the transnational arena and which norms can lay claim to de-facto validity. As long as there is no international demos or global public sphere where in-depth deliberations can take place and compromises be secured, fragmentation may remain the rule, which in turn provides opportunities for forum shopping for patients, brokers, doctors and medical managers alike.

Conclusion: Good Governance of Medical Tourism in a Globalised World

Prospects for regulation are not, however, so bleak. Instead of deploring a 'race to the bottom' or turning to political abstinence, it must be emphasised that regulation *is* possible. At least consensus on minimum standards can be achieved. It is the impetus of this chapter to assert that high minimum standards must be set and that international regulation must strive to raise these standards over time. At this point it also seems to be important to stress that moral pluralism must not mean moral relativism or that tolerance means not paying respect (Westacott, 2012). Claiming that we should not impose our values on other societies must not be used as a means to justify practices which, on reflection, are considered abusive or exploitative. Certain norms and values can be recognised as cutting across ethnicity, culture, geography and citizenship. Even though the interpretation of universal norms and rights can and will be pluralistic, consensus about some normative principles can and will be achieved internationally. In consequence, as a response to medical tourism, *the setting and heightening of international minimum standards* is a legitimate policy goal worth striving for. Governance and regulation thus should not be restricted to the least common denominator but must strive for progressively upgraded protection for patients, improved quality of care and responsible normative rules and practices. Hence, any regulatory framework that would be politically endorsed and implemented should be historically informed about segregation, discrimination and medical abuse; as such 'memory work' provides important lessons for the future. It should take a human rights-based approach and, thereby, necessarily be sensitive to gender, 'race', class, disability and other forms of socio-economic marginalisation, stigmatisation and exclusion. Such a commitment to a human rights framework rather than to free trade can be underlined in respective preambles to recommendations or regulatory texts.

This chapter has summarised horizontal and vertical means of governing medical tourism. It has highlighted regional and global agreements, conventions and court law as instruments that can be employed in good governance practices. It has issued a plea for high quality and responsible normative standards for regulating cross-border health care. As a preliminary conclusion, there is light at the end of the tunnel. Neither individuals nor collectives are helpless when it comes to governing medical tourism. At times, foreign pressures can be supportive in breaking taboos, and abuses can be prevented by publicity. Medical tourism involves risks, but it may also create opportunities for constitutionalisation in the international realm and for the establishment of valid norms borne out of normative contestations. A multiplicity of actors, state and non-state, private as well as public are involved in such ongoing struggles. It is the duty of practitioners as well as academics not only to shed light on practices and processes, to provide evidence and to correct false assumptions but also to deliberate about implications, and last but not least, to help in the creation of good governance practices.

References

Bubela, T. and Caulfield, T., 2004. Do the Print Media 'Hype' Genetic Research? A comparison of newspaper stories and peer-reviewed research papers. *Canadian Medical Association Journal*, 170(9), pp. 1,399–407.

Caulfield, T. and Condit, C., 2012. Science and the Sources of Hype. *Public Health Genomics*, 15(3–4), pp. 209–17.

Cohen, I.G., 2010. Medical Tourism: The view from 10,000 feet. *Hastings Center Report*, 40(2), pp. 11–12.

Council of Europe, 2012. *Towards a Council of Europe Convention to Combat Trafficking in Organs, Tissues and Cells of Human Origin.* Doc. 13082. 20 December. [online] Available at: <http://assembly.coe.int/ASP/XRef/X2H-DW-XSL.asp?fileid=19236&lang=EN> [Accessed 29 December 2013].

Crooks, V., Kingsbury, P., Snyder, J. and Johnston, R., 2010. What is Known about the Patient's Experience of Medical Tourism? A scoping review. *BMC Health Services Research*, 10(1), p. 266.

de Arellano, A.B.R., 2007. Patients Without Borders: The emergence of medical tourism. *International Journal of Health Services*, 37(1), 193–8.

Delmonico, F.L., 2009. The Implications of Istanbul Declaration on Organ Trafficking and Transplant Tourism. *Current Opinion on Organ Transplantation*, 14(2), pp. 116–19.

European Commission, 2006. *Report on the Regulation of Reproductive Cell Donation in the European Union. Results of survey.* Brussels: European Commission.

Fisher, E., Jones, J. and von Schomberg, R., eds, 2006. *Implementing the Precautionary Principle: Perspectives and Prospects.* Cheltenham: Edward Elgar.

Hoffmann-Riem, W., 2000. *Rechtswissenschaftliche Innovationsforschung als Reaktion auf gesellschaftlichen Innovationsbedarf.* [online] Available at: <http://www2.jura.uni-hamburg.de/ceri/publ/download01.PDF> [Accessed 28 February 2013].

Hyder, N., 2013. India Limits Surrogacy Visas to Married Couples. *BioNews*, 689, 21 January. [online] Available at: <http://www.bionews.org.uk/page_242618.asp> [Accessed 29 December 2013].

Johnston, R., Crooks, V., Snyder, J. and Kingsbury, P., 2010. What is Known about the Effects of Medical Tourism in Destination and Departure Countries? A scoping review. *International Journal for Equity in Health*, 9(1), p. 24. [online] Available at: <http://www.equityhealthj.com/content/9/1/24> [Accessed 29 December 2013].

Keller, M., 2013. Herz auf Bestellung. *Die Zeit.* [online] Available at: <http://www.zeit.de/2013/11/China-Transplantationen-Organhandel> [Accessed 29 December 2013].

Kulish, N. and Cottrell, C., 2012. German Health Care Attracts Foreign Patients. *The New York Times.* [online] Available at: <http://www.nytimes.

com/2012/12/21/world/europe/german-health-care-attracts-foreign-patients. html?_r=0> [Accessed 29 December 2013].

Lunt, N., Green, S.T., Mannion, R. and Horsfall, D., 2012a. Quality, Safety and Risk in Medical Tourism. In: M.C. Hall, ed. 2012. *Medical Tourism: The ethics, regulation, and marketing of health mobility*. London: Routledge, ch. 2.

Lunt, N., Mannion, R. and Exworthy, M., 2012b. A Framework for Exploring the Policy Implications of UK Medical Tourism and International Patient Flows. *Social Policy & Administration*, 47(1), pp. 1–25.

Lunt, N., Smith, R., Exworthy, M., Green, S.T., Horsfall, D. et al., 2011. *Medical Tourism: Treatments, markets and health system implications: A scoping review*. OECD. [online] Available at: <http://www.oecd.org/els/ healthpoliciesanddata/48723982.pdf> [Accessed 29 December 2013].

Magnus, D. and Cho, M.K., 2007. Therapeutic Misconception and Stem Cell Research. *Nature Reports Stem Cells*. [online] Available at: <http://www. nature.com/stemcells/2007/0709/070927/full/stemcells.2007.88.html> [Accessed 29 December 2013].

Mayntz, R., 1998. New Challenges to Governance Theory. *Jean Monet Chair Papers No.50*. [online] available at: <http://www.uned.es/113016/ docencia/spd%20-%20doctorado%202001–02/Introducci%F3n/Mayntz%20 governance%20EUI%201998.htm> [Accessed 29 December 2013].

O'Neill, O., 2002. *Autonomy and Trust in Bioethics*. Cambridge: Cambridge University Press.

Pocock, N.S. and Phua, K.H., 2011. Medical Tourism and Policy Implications for Health Systems: A conceptual framework from a comparative study of Thailand, Singapore and Malaysia. *Globalization and Health*, 7(12), pp. 1–12.

Pennings, G., 2002. Reproductive Tourism as Moral Pluralism in Motion. *Journal of Medical Ethics* 28(6), pp. 337–41.

Scharpf, F.W., 1997. *Games Real Actors Play: Actor-centered institutionalism in policy research*. Boulder, CO: Westview.

Schneider, I., 2003. 'Pro-Life' and 'Pro-Choice': Overcoming the misleading controversy. *Human Nature: A working conference on the challenges of the new human genetics technologies – within and beyond the limits of human nature*. Berlin, Germany, 12–15 October 2003. [online] Available at: <http:// www.docstoc.com/docs/159961388/Ingrid-Schneider-Pro-life-and-Pro-choice-Overcoming-the-Glow> [Accessed 29 December 2014].

———, 2009. Indirect Commodification of Ova Donation for Assisted Reproduction and for Human Cloning Research – Proposals for supranational regulation. In: M. Steinmann, P. Sykora and U. Wiesing, eds 2009. *Altruism Reconsidered*. Farnham and Burlington: Ashgate Publishing. pp. 209–41.

———, 2010. *The European Patent System: Shifts in Governance through Parliaments and Civil Society*. Frankfurt and New York: Campus.

———, 2014. The Body, the Law, and the Market: Public policy implications in a liberal state. In: M. Albers, T. Hoffmann and J. Reinhardt, eds, 2014. *Human Rights and Human Nature*. Dordrecht: Springer, pp. 197–215.

Stone-Sweet, A., 2011. Managing Difference: Constitutional pluralism and transnational rights protection. In: K. Raube and A. Sattler, eds, 2011. *Difference and Democracy.* Frankfurt and New York: Campus, pp. 227–44.

Tattara, G., 2010. Medical Tourism and Domestic Population Health. *University Ca'Foscari of Venice, Research Paper No. 02–10.* [online] Available at: <http://ssrn.com/abstract=1544224 or http://dx.doi.org/10.2139/ssrn.1544224> [Accessed 29 December 2013].

The Local, 2011. Surrogate Children Have No Right to German Passport, Court Rules. *The Local*, 28 April.

Westacott, E., 2012. Moral Relativism. *International Encyclopedia of Philosophy.* [online] Available at: <http://www.iep.utm.edu/moral-re/> [Accessed 29 December 2013].

Chapter 12

Dislodging the Direct-to-Consumer Marketing of Stem Cell-Based Interventions from Medical Tourism

Tamra Lysaght and Douglas Sipp

Introduction

Stem cells are the focus of an emergent field of clinical research and application that is frequently described as having enormous therapeutic potential. While currently only certain types of blood-forming (hematopoietic) stem cells are used routinely in the treatment of very specific types of blood and immune system disorders, many other proposed approaches are being investigated in clinical trials (Daley, 2012). For example, investigational products derived from human embryonic stem cells (hESCs) have entered clinical trials of uses in dry type age-related macular degeneration and spinal cord injuries, while foetal-derived cells are being tested for the rehabilitation of ischemic stroke patients (Mack, 2011). A number of large-scale efficacy trials with autologous bone-marrow-derived stem cells for the treatment of acute myocardial infarction have either been completed or are underway (Clifford et al., 2012). More than a thousand other registered clinical trials using both allogeneic and autologous sources of somatic (or 'adult') stem cells (ASC) are also underway (Li, Atkins and Bubela, 2013), although many of these focus on the use of hematopoietic stem cells for indications they are currently used to treat, such as lymphoma, leukaemia and auto-immune diseases (Daley, 2012).

Despite the vast majority of proposed stem cell-based approaches remaining in the early phases of clinical trials, an alarming number of interventions using what are claimed to be stem cells or stem cell-based products are being offered to patients on a commercial basis outside the standard of care. These stem cell-based interventions (SCBI) are typically marketed direct to the consumer (DTC) via the Internet, and are often targeted at an improbably wide range of diseases and illnesses, including cardiovascular diseases, Down syndrome, liver disease, Parkinson's disease, HIV/AIDS, Alzheimer's disease, cerebral palsy, autism and multiple sclerosis (Lau et al., 2008; Regenberg et al., 2009). In this chapter, we refer to this commercial activity as the *direct-to-consumer marketing of stem cell-based interventions* (DTC-SCBI). In adopting this term, we must emphasise that what unifies such companies is the use of the term 'stem cells' in their marketing and promotional materials; it does not indicate that the products and services they advertise in fact contain or make use of actual human stem cells. We also note that, for reasons outlined in this chapter, this label de-emphasises and shifts the focus from the consumers (patients) to the suppliers (clinics), although for the sake of convenience we occasionally use the term to refer to the set of actors on both sides of the supply–demand interaction.

While one recent systematic review indicated that certain types of SCBI are well tolerated (Lalu et al., 2012), evidence of efficacy remains scant and, with the exception of the Korea Food and Drug Administration in South Korea, no authority responsible for the regulation of cell and tissue-based products in a major industrialised country has authorised a stem cell biologic drug for the market (Park, 2012). Many companies that advertise 'stem cell' interventions therefore generally operate in countries that are either unable or unwilling to monitor their claims and activities (Kiatpongsan and Sipp, 2009). In the past decade, international travel by patients seeking DTC-SCBI that are unavailable in their home countries has become increasingly common.

In the fields of bioethics, social science, and medicine, scholars have often placed this phenomenon within the broader category of medical travel, which is colloquially known as 'medical tourism', and the label 'stem cell tourism' has entered the popular and professional discourses in reflection of this sub-categorisation. At first glance, DTC-SCBI shares some evident characteristics with activities that are broadly associated with businesses that cater to patients seeking medical care abroad; that is, they involve patients seeking medical care beyond the borders of their home country, and healthcare providers in foreign countries who market their services DTC. However, scholars have also recognised that while the DTC-SCBI phenomenon bears some relevance to the broader field, it lies at the periphery of what constitutes medical travel, as an extreme activity that is more typically likened with patients travelling to access morally contestable activities, such as abortion, euthanasia, and organ transplantation or to receive interventions that lack solid scientific support. In the following chapter, we take this position further by arguing that DTC-SCBI differs categorically from other forms of medical travel or tourism because:

1. Medical tourism represents the standard of care in medicine, whereas DTC-SCBI does not;
2. The term 'tourism' misrepresents the activities of clinics offering DTC-SCBI domestically and misplaces the focus of attention onto patients rather than providers;
3. The term 'stem cell' misrepresents the poorly characterised cellular preparations that are delivered to patients and the documented cases of fraud in DTC-SCBI.

Before elaborating on this argument, we will first provide a brief outline of some recent literature that deals with the construct of 'medical tourism'.

The Conceptual Category Medical Tourism and DCT-SCBI

The term 'medical tourism' is generally used to describe a niche category of specialist travel in which medical services are marketed DTC and often in packages that can also include flights, hotels, sightseeing and other activities that are typically associated with the broader scope of 'tourism' (Connell, 2011). However, there is no universally accepted definition of medical tourism and the term is contested (Hall, 2011; Turner and Hodges, 2012). For some scholars, use of the term 'tourism' is problematic because it implies pleasurable, relaxing activities that are not generally associated with medicine and it blurs distinctions between desperately ill people travelling for live-saving procedures with more discretionary elective surgery (Whittaker, Manderson and Cartwright, 2010). For others, it is an industry-driven term that promotes a 'marketplace model that disregards the suffering that patients experience' (Kangas, 2010, p. 350) and 'insinuates leisurely travelling and does not capture the seriousness of most patient mobility' (Glinos et al., 2010, p. 1146). Thus, the term 'medical travel' is often used instead of 'medical tourism' even though an industry has emerged that identifies and markets itself as such.

Academic approaches also tend to focus on the international dimensions of medical travel. However, the flow of patients between source and destination countries may be more complex than the focus implies. While there is a lack of evidence that accurately gauges the numbers and movements of patients who engage in international travel for medical purposes (Lunt and Carrera, 2010), Connell (2011, p. x) identifies three main groups:

1. Patients travelling from more developed countries who are unable or unwilling to pay or endure long waiting times for medical procedures and are not part of the socioeconomic elite;
2. Patients who are part of the socioeconomic elite in developing countries where medical standards are poor and seek high quality care elsewhere;
3. Diaspora travellers seeking treatment in countries of origin, which are thought to make up the majority of medical travel.

Connell (2011) also suggests that the majority of medical travel is regional (for example, patients travelling within Asia or within Europe) rather than transcontinental journeys. Meanwhile, domestic suppliers in the United States have begun to compete with overseas markets by, for example, offering lower hospital fees for price-sensitive patients willing to travel for a cheaper deal (Hudson and Li, 2011). However, it is unclear what, if any, implications domestic supply has for an analytical category that is focused on the international movement of patients.

Furthermore, the category is defined by patients travelling to access some form of medical treatment (Lunt and Carrera, 2010). Distinguishing travel for the purpose of accessing medical services from other health-related and wellbeing activities can be challenging, however, particularly as the meaning of these terms can vary across different cultures and countries (Hall, 2013). Generally speaking, medical travel includes dental and cosmetic procedures, surgical interventions and infertility treatments. Yet some scholars have excluded travel for access to pharmaceutical drugs and medicines that are cheaper elsewhere while others exclude complementary medicines (Connell, 2011), presumably on the basis that they do not constitute 'medicine'. Others have argued that medical tourism should also exclude illegal and unethical activities such as organ transplantation (Turner, 2008). Given the seriousness of the *medical indications* that many patients are travelling with when seeking an interventions with DCT-SCBI, we argue that similar rationale can apply to the exclusion of DTC-SCBI from the category of medical tourism.

DTC-SCBI Does Not Represent the Standard of Care in Medicine

The constellation of activities undertaken by patients and consumers grouped within the conceptual framework of 'medical tourism' share two common features: international travel and therapy-seeking. The term medical tourism, however, is also used more broadly to refer not only to these activities, but also to the network of providers that has emerged to serve the demand for such medical services, including hospitals and clinics, patient brokers, travel services, marketing and advertising. In this wider sense, medical tourism describes not only a form of consumer activity but the industry as a whole, encompassing both the demand and the supply sides of the equation. In many countries this industry represents a significant source of national economic activity, and is supported by government incentives for local businesses and regulated as any other economic activity. Private agencies and industry organisations provide further industry-oriented services, such as accreditation, training, lobbying and holding of conferences to promote standards and showcase new developments. Thus, the medical tourism industry is an increasingly well-developed industry sector, comprising consumers, providers, local and national governments and various ancillary organisations.

As the medical tourism industry has matured, it has engaged in activities to solidify and protect its identity, and exclude from its self-definition actors and behaviours that would potentially harm or confuse its reputation. Notably, this boundary work is coordinated primarily by supply-side industry members, not by consumers. As with many maturing industries, this work emphasises coordination, cooperation and compliance with regulatory authorities, to ensure that regulations are developed in a way that promotes (or at least does not harm) the interests of the industry. The medical tourism industry has particularly striven, with varying success, to develop and maintain standards for medical care, as a key feature of the self-image the industry has sought to cultivate is quality of care: patients are encouraged to perceive the standard of care at international providers to be as good as, or superior to, that which is readily available in their home countries. There are of course examples of medical tourism hospitals offering sub-standard care, squandering patient resources or wasting their money, but medical tourism as an industry is careful to hold these up as non-normative examples.

It is thus interesting and instructive to examine how the medical tourism industry, perceives DTC-SCBI. The US-based Medical Tourism Association has cautioned members about the problem of unlicensed stem cell treatments, citing safety and accountability concerns (Stephano and Abratt, 2012). In a similar vein, the largest medical tourism hospital in Thailand, Bumrungrad International Hospital (2009), has published a statement of policy on its website that specifically states its position on the delivery of stem cell interventions that have not passed regulatory scrutiny or entered standard of care:

> We will develop capabilities and offer such treatments to our patients when they are accepted by the international medical community. If our clinical research program does participate in any trials, we assure our patients of the following:
> - the experimental nature of the treatment will be clearly explained;
> - we will adhere to guidelines of the Thai FDA and Medical Council, even if such guidelines are not yet official law; and
> - we will not attempt to profit from experimental treatments not yet proven.

Subsequent to the statement from Bumrungrad, the Thai Medical Council published guidelines on stem cell clinical research and development, requiring approval from the Council for clinical studies and uses of stem cells (Sipp, 2009). The emphasis on international community standards, even in the absence of a national regulatory framework governing the introduction of new stem cell products and procedures is telling.

Regulators and governments, including many that strongly support the development of the medical tourism sector, have also sought to differentiate DTC-SCBI from 'legitimate' medical tourism. Regulatory agencies, health ministries and national medical councils in a great many countries have issued public warnings on the risks of 'stem cell tourism' or threatened action against companies engaged in marketing such services. In some instances, however, there has been an apparent lack of coordination across agencies within a single country, resulting in conflicting agendas.

A few examples illustrate how bodies with a primarily economic remit may work at cross-purposes to those engaged in ensuring quality medical care. The Thailand Board of Investment (2008) granted incentives to DTC-SCBI firm Theravitae prior to the development of national regulations, and even after the Thai Medical Council announced rules intended to rein in the industry, a website maintained by the Tourism Authority of Thailand provided links to a number of hospitals and clinics offering unlicensed stem cell interventions on its Thailand Medical Tourism Portal (Tourism Authority of Thailand, 2012). Similarly, in China, hospitals operated on a commercial basis by the military have escaped regulation of their DTC-SCBI businesses by the Ministry of Health and State Food and Drug Administration, thanks to a separate regulatory system in place for hospitals operated by the People's Liberation Army. These cases, however, are the exception to the rule of increased oversight and regulation of SCBI that do not meet the international medical community's standards of care.

As with many business sectors in a globalised world, the medical tourism industry includes many entities that operate in multiple countries – such businesses enjoy certain advantages with respect to government regulation in that their activities may extend beyond the jurisdictional reach of any single nation, and in many cases are free to seek out favourable regulatory venues (regulatory shopping or arbitrage), which can be used as leverage in bargaining with governments seeking the economic benefits of a strong medical tourism sector. But the centrality of the quality of care to the medical tourism's self-promoted identity generally prevents companies from flouting regulations or seeking out countries in which regulations are absent or insufficient. In the case of DTC-SCBI, however, vendors tend to develop in, or seek out, those nations in which relevant laws are lacking or unenforced. At present, South Korea is the only country in which stem cell products other than those intended for established uses of hematopoietic stem cells in the treatment of blood and immune conditions have received market authorisation (Park, 2012).

An important component in the marketing strategies of companies engaging in DTC-SCBI is how they frame their interventions not as the standard of care, but as 'experimental treatments'. This framing is also grossly misleading. Patients travelling great distances for DTC-SCBI may see themselves as 'pilgrims' on a quest 'to obtain an experimental treatment unavailable elsewhere in the world' (Song, 2010, p. 386), yet the practices of the clinics they visit do not constitute medical research or experimental medicine. Medical research is a highly structured activity that is designed to test hypotheses and produce generalisable knowledge. According to internationally-accepted standards for medical research espoused in the *Declaration of Helsinki*, protocols should be subject to independent review by an ethics committee and 'must conform to generally accepted scientific principles, be based on a thorough knowledge of the scientific literature … and adequate laboratory and, as appropriate, animal experimentation' (World Medical Association, 2000). As an academic field of medical research committed to scientific principles of clinical investigation, experimental medicine in no way resembles the activities of operators involved in DTC-SCBI.

As part of clinical practice, licensed medical practitioners are provided with a degree of discretion in departing from accepted practices or varying the standard of care in order to suit the needs of individual patients. International guidance permits this type of 'experimentation', often given another misleading label of 'innovation', but only under highly exceptional circumstances. According to the Declaration of Helsinki, medical interventions that lie outside the standard of care may be administered to small patient populations as a life-saving measure where existing treatments are ineffective or non-existent (World Medical Association, 2000). However, the document also states that: 'Where possible, this intervention should be made the object of research, designed to evaluate its safety and efficacy.

In all cases, new information should be recorded and, where appropriate, made publicly available'.

The Guidelines of the International Society for Stem Cell Research (ISSCR, 2008, p. 15) also allow for highly exceptional circumstances in which:[1]

> Clinician-scientists may provide unproven stem cell-based interventions to at most a very small number of patients outside the context of a formal clinical trial, provided that:
>
> a) there is a written plan for the procedure that includes ... scientific rationale and justification explaining why the procedure has a reasonable chance of success, including any preclinical evidence of proof-of- principle for efficacy and safety ...
>
> b) the written plan is approved through a peer review process by appropriate experts who have no vested interest in the proposed procedure.

Additionally, the ISSCR guidance (2008, p. 5) distinguishes between these 'legitimate attempts at medical innovation' and the 'commercial purveyance of unproven stem cell interventions' where 'a large series of patients' are administered with stem cells 'outside a clinical trial' and charged for such services. Providers of DTC-SCBI are, in many cases, clearly falling within this latter category of 'commercial purveyance'. As their activities can be neither categorised as medical practice, experimental medicine or research, they ought to be excluded from a conceptual construct based on an industry that strives to provide only the standard of care.

'Tourism' is Patient-Centric and Misrepresents the Domestic Trade in DCT-SCBI

A broad range of stem cell products are regulated as biologic drugs in many nations, which effectively precludes the entry of unlicensed stem cell interventions into these markets. In other countries, the regulatory status of certain types of stem cell interventions, typically those involving the use of autologous ASCs, has been more ambiguous. In the United States, for example, many clinics have marketed interventions using putative stem cell-derived products from autologous adipose tissue or bone marrow, with the contention that such interventions are minimally manipulated, homologous uses, and/or delivered as part of the same surgical procedure and therefore do not fall under the federal laws regulating the manufacture of human cell and tissue products (HCT/P). However, the FDA has issued warning letters in a number of such cases, and a US District Court upheld the FDA's jurisdiction against a challenge from one such company in

---

1   At the time of writing, these Guidelines were undergoing review and may have been revised since publication.

2012 (Cyranoski, 2012), suggesting that the legal validity of these claims may be precarious. A number of companies have also sought market entry for point of care cell processing devices via the 510(k) pathway, which allows for devices to be cleared for market without testing in human subjects if it can be shown that there is a significantly equivalent predicate device already on the market. Importantly, this enables licensed physicians to use such devices in manners other than the approved use. As a result of such claims and practices, ostensible SCBI are now commonly available in several US states and marketed DTC.

One clear impact of this global regulatory patchwork and local challenges to the extent of relevant laws has been that clinics now operate in a great many countries around the world, from developing nations to several of the world's most economically advanced countries. For this reason, it is no longer necessary for many patients to seek stem cell treatments outside their home countries. However, given that the interventions on offer, which are frequently in areas of aesthetic plastic surgery or orthopaedic medicine, have not been validated by rigorous clinical testing, authorised for marketing by a competent authority, or been accepted as standard of care by the broader medical community, it is clear that what has previously been referred to as stem cell 'tourism' no longer requires international travel by patients.

A second, perhaps more critical problem with the use of 'tourism' to refer to patients seeking out putative stem cell treatment is that this descriptor focuses squarely on the patients, rather than the providers (for it is the patients who undertake the travelling or 'tourism'). To start with, there is evidence to suggest that patients seeking out DTC-SCBI abroad do not engage in the types of sightseeing or convalescent activities that are generally associated with 'medical tourism' (Song, 2010). From Song's (2010, p. 386) anthropological study of patients who had travelled to China, this categorisation was viewed as trivialising their motivations and experiences: 'Marketing their experience as "medical tourism" misconstrues both the purpose and the significance of their journeys. Far from being a vacation on the cheap, these quests for a cure involve significant expense and hardship'.

Furthermore, as outlined above, an industry comprising primary providers, as well as recruitment and brokering services, and various activities (*soi-disant* professional and organisations, private foundations, NPOs, etc.) has emerged not only to answer, but to cultivate, patient demand for such services. Similarly, the vast majority of criticism of the 'stem cell tourism' phenomenon has been directed at commercial actors, not at patients. Thus, scientists, physicians, media outlets, academic societies and patient advocacy groups who call attention to the risks and problems associated with DTC-SCBI should take care in choosing their targets. If, as we believe, many 'stem cell' clinics are aggressively marketing sub-optimal care direct to patients, often in contravention to local laws and international medical standards, the 'tourists' are victims, not perpetrators.

'Stem Cells' May Misrepresent What Is Provided to Patients

If we can eliminate the 'tourism' from the practice of DTC-SCBI, what of the term 'stem cells'? Looking at marketing claims and legal developments, it becomes clear that in a number of cases companies have used the term 'stem cells' to advertise products or services that do not contain bona fide stem cells. Perhaps the most common example of this are practices that market various forms of 'live cells' or *Frischzellen*, which are preparations of tissues from foetal animals, such as sheep or rabbits. This practice dates back at least to the 1920s, and has seen a recent revival that coincides with the excitement surrounding 'stem cell therapies' – indeed, many clinics now advertise their freeze-dried xenogeneic foetal tissue preparations as if these are stem cell products, when it is unclear that these products contain or act on human stem cells in any meaningful way. Several cases have also been reported in which people associated with companies advertising 'stem cell treatments' have been discovered to be fraudulently delivering something different altogether. In the UK, one physician was found to be injecting his 'stem cell' patients with bovine cells intended for laboratory use (Ward, 2010).

More generally, however, the state of science in stem cell biology has not yet progressed to the point at which even leading scientists agree on fundamental questions such as the properties (gene expression, surface proteins, epigenetic modifications, etc.) and functions that characterise specific types of stem cells. While a consensus appears to have emerged on the characterisation of hematopoietic stem cells, which have been in clinical use for decades, for other stem cell types, such as neural stem cells, mesenchymal stem cells (MSCs), embryonic stem cells (ESCs) and induced pluripotent stem cells (iPSCs), the picture is less clear. A working group organised by the International Society for Cell Therapy explicitly recognised this in a position paper on MSCs, concluding that at the time of writing there was insufficient evidence to justify the term 'mesenchymal stem cells' and proposing 'multipotent mesenchymal stromal cells' as an alternative (Dominici et al., 2006). This is a centrally important distinction, as the vast majority of so-called stem cell interventions marketed DTC over the Internet claim to use or affect MSCs from various tissue sources (bone marrow, peripheral blood, perinatal tissue, adipose tissue, etc.).

Conclusions

While DTC-SCBI intuitively belongs within the broader category of medical tourism, there are particular aspects of this phenomenon that makes its inclusion within this category problematic. From the above, we can see that not only is the use of 'tourism' inappropriate in many cases of DTC-SCBI, but that 'stem cell' is also in question. The umbrella term 'stem cell tourism' appears to be inadequate to cover the full range of commercial activities that it is currently used to refer to. The interventions being offered to patients also lie well outside the standard of care and, indeed, bear little resemblance to the practice of medicine. Thus, the uncritical annexing of DTC-SCBI as medical tourism not only masks and prevents a more nuanced understanding of the issues at stake, it may inadvertently legitimate ethically dubious, if not illegal, activities that constitute as neither medicine or experimental research.

While we acknowledge that the term 'stem cell tourism' is a catchy rhetorical device and is likely to remain in the popular discourse in the foreseeable future, we would also encourage scholars in this area to take greater care with the language used to portray the activities of patients and providers of DTC-SCBI. Analogising DTC-SCBI with providers of international medical services may have unwarranted legitimation effects for practitioners who establish businesses based on interventions with poorly characterised cellular preparations that lack credible evidence of efficacy, or worse, fraudsters posing as physicians selling nothing but saline injections. The analogy with medical tourism also misplaces the focus of attention on patients when it should be on the medical professionals that engage in these activities. This patient-centric tourism approach disguises the serious underlying issues around the regulation and governance of professional behaviour and clinical research, which should actually be the focus of critical discussion on this matter.

Future efforts in gathering more empirical evidence on DTC-SCBI should ensure that service providers meet some basic requirements before being categorised as being part of the medical tourism industry. First, websites offering DTC-SCBI should represent a legitimate organisation, institution or company (that is, one that is legally registered as such with relevant authorities and possesses associated tax file numbers, etc.), and that any medical practitioners named on the site are fully licensed and registered to practice medicine in the jurisdiction in which they operate. Second, providers of DTC-SCBI should be able to offer assurances of quality and evidence that the cellular preparations being administered to patients actually contain stem cells (that is, the organisation or institution should be registered with the relevant authorities that regulate good tissue practices the local competent authority, as is the case in many countries for other biological products, including blood products, gametes and other cell and tissue products). Third, research in this area should also distinguish between organisations and institutions that are trying to provide the standard of care from those that are only offering interventions that lack evidence of efficacy and are not part of a supervised clinical trial.

References

Bumrungrad International Hospital, 2009. Stem Cell Treatment. [online] Available at: <http://www.bumrungrad.com/overseas-medical-care/medical-services/ info/stemcell.aspx> [Accessed 29 January 2013].

Clifford, D.M., Fisher, S.A., Brunskill, S.J., Doree, C., Mathur, A. et al., 2012. Long-Term Effects of Autologous Bone Marrow Stem Cell Treatment in Acute Myocardial Infarction: Factors that may influence outcomes. *PLoS ONE*, 7(5), p. e37373.

Connell, J., 2011. *Medical Tourism*. Wallingford: CAB International.

Cyranoski, D., 2012. FDA's Claims Over Stem Cells Upheld. *Nature*, 488(7,409), p. 14.

Daley, G.Q., 2012. The Promise and Perils of Stem Cell Therapeutics. *Cell Stem Cell*, 10(6), pp. 740–49.

Dominici, M., Le Blanc, K., Mueller, I., Slaper-Cortenbach, I., Marini, F. et al., 2006. Minimal Criteria for Defining Multipotent Mesenchymal Stromal Cells. The International Society for Cellular Therapy position statement. *Cytotherapy*, 8(4), pp. 315–17.

Glinos, I.A., Baeten, R., Helble, M. and Maarse, H., 2010. A Typology of cross-Border Patient Mobility. *Health and Place*, 16(6), pp. 1,145–55.

Hall, M.C., 2011. Health and Medical Tourism: A kill or cure for global public health? *Tourism Review*, 66(1/2), pp. 4–15.

———, 2013. Medical and Health Tourism: The development and implications of medicla mobility. In: M.C. Hall, ed., 2013. *Medical Tourism: The ethics, regulation, and marketing of health mobility*. New York: Routledge. pp. 3–28.

Hudson, S. and Li, X., 2011. Domestic Medical Tourism: A neglected dimension of medical tourism research. *Journal of Hospitality Marketing and Management*, 21(3), pp. 227–46.

International Society for Stem Cell Research, 2008. *Guidelines for the Clinical Translation of Stem Cells*.[online]Available at: <http://www.isscr.org/clinical_trans/pdfs/ISSCRGLClinicalTrans.pdf> [Accessed 29 December 2013].

Kangas, B., 2010. Traveling for Medical Care in a Global World. *Medical Anthropology*, 29(4), pp. 344–62.

Kiatpongsan, S. and Sipp, D., 2009. Monitoring and Regulating Offshore Stem Cell Clinics. *Science*, 323(5,921), pp. 1,564–5.

Lalu, M.M., McIntyre, L., Pugliese, C., Fergusson, D., Winston, B.W. et al., 2012. Safety of Cell Therapy with Mesenchymal Stromal Cells (Safecell): A systematic review and meta-analysis of clinical trials. *PLoS ONE*, 7(10), p. e47559.

Lau, D., Ogbogu, U., Taylor, B., Stafinski, T., Menon, D. et al., 2008. Stem Cell Clinics Online: The direct-to-consumer portrayal of stem cell medicine. *Cell Stem Cell*, 3(6), pp. 591–4.

Li, M.D., Atkins, H. and Bubela, T. 2013. The global landscape of stem cell clinical trials. *Regenerative Medicine*, 9(1), pp. 27–39.

Lunt, N. and Carrera, P., 2010. Medical Tourism: Assessing the evidence on treatment abroad. *Maturitas*, 66(1), pp. 27–32.

Mack, G.S., 2011. ReNeuron and StemCells Get Green Light for Neural Stem Cell Trials. *Nature Biotechnology*, 29(2), pp. 95–7.

Park, S.B., 2012. South Korea Steps Up Stem-Cell Work. *Nature*. [online] Available at: <www.nature.com/news/south-korea-steps-up-stem-cell-work-1.10565> [Accessed 29 December 2013].

Regenberg, A.C., Hutchinson, L.A., Schanker, B. and Mathews, D.J.H., 2009. Medicine on the Fringe: Stem cell-based interventions in advance of evidence. *Stem Cells*, 27(9), pp. 2,312–19.

Sipp, D., 2009. The Rocky Road to Regulation. [10.1038/stemcells.2009.125]. *Nature Reports Stem Cells*. [online] Available at: <http://www.nature.com/stemcells/2009/0909/090923/full/stemcells.2009.125.html> [Accessed 29 December 2013].

Song, P. , 2010. Biotech Pilgrims and the Transnational Quest for Stem Cell Cures. *Medical Anthropology*, 29(4), pp. 384–402.

Stephano, R.-M. and Abratt, D., 2012. Restricting Unapproved Stem Cell Therapies – The persisting battle. *Medical Tourism Magazine*. [online] Available at: <http://medicaltourismmag.com/restricting-unapproved-stem-cell-therapies-the-persisting-battle/> [Accessed 29 December 2013].

Thailand Board of Investment, 2008. Thailand Moves Biotechnology Forward. *Thailand Investment Review*, 18(5), pp. 5–6.

Tourism Authority of Thailand, 2012. ThaiMedTourism.com. [online] Available at: <http://www.thailandmedtourism.com> [Accessed 29 January 2013].

Turner, L., 2008. 'Medical Tourism' Initiatives Should Exclude Commercial Organ Transplantation. *Journal of the Royal Society of Medicine*, 101(8), pp. 391–4.

Turner, L. and Hodges, J.R., 2012. Introduction: Health care goes global. In: J.R. Hodges, L. Turner and A.M. Kimball, eds, 2012. *Risks and Challenges in Medical Tourism: Understanding the global market for health services*. Santa Barbara, CA: Praeger, pp. 1–16.

Ward, V., 2010. Stem cell doctor Robert Trossel struck off medical register. *The Daily Telegraph*, [online] Available at: <http://www.telegraph.co.uk/health/healthnews/8033130/Stem-cell-doctor-Robert-Trossel-struck-off-medical-register.html> [Accessed 7 May 2012].

Whittaker, A., Manderson, L. and Cartwright, E., 2010. Patients Without Borders: Understanding medical travel. *Medical Anthropology*, 29(4), pp. 336–43.

World Medical Association, 2000. Declaration of Helsinki: Ethical principles for medical research involving human subjects. [online] Available at: <http://www.wma.net/en/30publications/10policies/b3/> [Accessed 23 May 2011].

Index

Page numbers in **bold** refer to figures and tables.